THE TEN
GUIDING LIGHTS

THE TEN
GUIDING LIGHTS
WORKBOOK

Etta Dale Hornsteiner

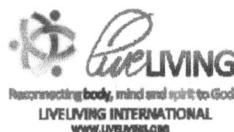

LIVE LIVING
Reconnecting **body**, mind and spirit to God
LIVE LIVING INTERNATIONAL
WWW.LIVELIVING.COM

Contents

Introduction

Principles are important because they guide us. They determine the decisions we make; and when they become our convictions, we live life passionately. In 2008, the Holy Spirit directed me to write a health and wellness Bible study using the Ten Commandments given to Moses and the Ancient Hebrews. He revealed to me principles within these commandments that would be the foundation for developing a healthy and fit life. For me, this revelation was exciting, because it was the missing link I had been seeking as a personal trainer.

After 13 years of teaching high school, I left the educational system to pursue a career in fitness, which had become my passion while competing in amateur bodybuilding competitions. However, as I trained my clients, I realized something was not connecting. My clients were struggling to make lifestyle changes without any truths that were bigger than they. Being accountable to a truth or living with a conviction provides a foundation. As believers, this foundation is the Word of God. Our guide to living a healthy and fit life is the Bible. As citizens of the kingdom of God, we live by its mandate. We are obligated to respond to its teachings with obedience, and this obedience is out of love—not guilt, fear or coercion. Hence, we are no longer led by our bodies but by our spirits' desire to please God—our taste buds do not rule us and neither do we listen to our bodies when they tell us not to exercise. We obey the voice of the Holy Spirit. Oh, how wonderful life would be if this were truly happening!

Instead, we struggle in our walk of faith because of the lack of discipline shown in our lives physically, mentally and spiritually. *The Ten Guiding Lights to Health and Wholeness* is intended to encourage us to reunite the three dimensions of our being—body, mind and spirit—in order to maximize our life experience here on earth—to live life to the fullest as Jesus exhorted in John 10:10. These three entities cannot exist in isolation from each other. They must be united and governed by the Word of God. This study, therefore, requires us to make the Word of God a priority. Doesn't the scripture command us to seek the kingdom of God *first*, and then all other things will be *added*? Ironically, that includes weight loss, whether it is physical, emotional or spiritual.

This 12-week Bible study is a transformational journey, involving mind, body and spirit. On this journey, you will be required to bring the following items:

- **The Bible** –Unless otherwise noted, the *New Living Translation* is mainly used in this study.

- **Journal Notebook** – You will be asked to reflect and write. The Holy Spirit will speak to you on paper. Some revelations will be pleasant; some might be shocking; some might be epiphanies. The point is the journal writing must be approached seriously and not pushed to the side.

- **Life's Experiences (Activities)** – The success of this study is based on you. The result is proportionate to the effort you invest. The "applications" are not *optional* assignments to the weekly lessons. They will help in bringing about lasting changes.

- **Food Journal** – Research has shown that people who keep a food journal are much more successful than others in losing and maintaining weight loss. Although this is not a weight-loss program per se, a food journal is encouraged in order to foster a healthy lifestyle.

- **Meditation** – Learning to sit still in the presence of God will be practiced in this study.

Living a healthy life means to be whole—healthy in our body, mind and spirit. To experience this *wholeness* that Christ has already given to us, we may have to uproot old ways of thinking that have set us up for failure and implement principles that guarantee success. Ephesians 4:22-23 (AMPC) emphasizes the importance of this transformation:

> Strip yourselves of your former nature [put off and discard your old unrenewed self] which characterized your previous manner of life and becomes corrupt through lusts and desires that spring from delusion;

> And be constantly renewed in the spirit of your mind [having a fresh mental and spiritual attitude].

The kingdom of God is about establishing God's rulership on Earth over our body, mind and spirit. His rulership requires a new way of thinking, feeling and living as we journey.

Check to make sure you have everything you need to succeed on this journey.

All the best,
Etta Dale Hornsteiner

Chapter 1

Avoid Addictions

"You must not have any other god but me."

Goals:

Develop a holistic attitude toward health and wellness

Become aware of my body as God's kingdom within

Understand how my health and wellness relates to God's kingdom message

Understand how the first commandment protects and restores my health and well being

Objectives:

Recognize foods to avoid

State the purpose of my body

Explain the spiritual impact of addiction

Recognize God's purpose for pleasure

Identify God's mandate for my life

Recognize the importance of physical and spiritual health

Extend the metaphor of the body as the temple of God to the kingdom of God within

Choose one of the following goals above to focus on for the week

Your goal for this week:

_____

_____

"It is said that the brain wants the very substance that is doing it the most harm. In truth, we cannot trust our own brains to do what is best for us."[1] Instead, we have to remind and retrain ourselves by first understanding the original intent of our design as spiritual beings within a body.

The ventral tegmental area (VTA)—the "reward" system—of the brain manufactures the neurotransmitter dopamine. Dopamine is released "in anticipation of meeting drives (like eating, drinking, and sex), in response to pain, and has been thought to underlie the feelings of pleasure."[2] Unfortunately, some people become addicted to dopamine and dependent on the substance that trigger it.

1. Read Colossian 1: 16. Dopamine is a neurotransmitter responsible for feelings of pleasure. Do you think God created the neurotransmitter dopamine? If so, what do you think was His purpose for creating it?

_____

_____

_____

2. What happens when we become dependent on feelings of pleasure?

_____

_____

_____

3. Why is an addiction considered a god?

_____

_____

_____

4. According to Revelation 4:11, why did God create us?

_____

_____

Dr. Myles Munroe, author of *Rediscovering the Kingdom: Ancient Hope for Our 21st Century World*, reminds us that "[w]here purpose is not known, abuse is inevitable."[3] The body's ultimate purpose is for God, not for food, drugs or sex. When we contemplate this principle, we begin to see the body as the possession we should keep sacred for the pleasure of God.[4] Worship in the body becomes a way of pleasing God. Discipline of the body becomes a way to offer our bodies as living sacrifice. We are cautioned to "guard against our base desires, because death is stationed near the gateway of pleasure."[5] Too much pleasure makes us dull; too much food slows us down; too much alcohol turns us into fools, and too much television/Internet turns us into living zombies.

5. What is the purpose of the body?

_____

_____

_____

6. Explain the quote, "Where purpose is not known abuse is inevitable".

_____

_____

7. How does the quote above explain how we can become vulnerable to addictions?

_____

_____

8. Explain Romans 12:1. How are we to present our bodies?

_____

_____

_____

9. How is discipline like a "sacrifice"?

_____

_____

_____

10. Galatians 5:22-23 says, "But the Holy Spirit produces this kind of fruit in our lives: love, joy, peace, patience, kindness, goodness, faithfulness, gentleness and self-control. Against such things there is no law." Circle the word in the scripture that is the closest in meaning to "dominion".

11. Our dominion mandate can be found in Genesis 1:28. Write out this mandate.

_____

_____

_____

12. How is this mandate relevant to our health and wellness?

_____

_____

_____

13. Most of us want to look and feel good and to live a long life, seeing not only our children grow up but also their offspring as well. Although all of these are good, what ultimately should be the real reason for being healthy and well? In the biblical context, why is it important to pay attention to the body by caring for it?

_____

_____

_____

14. My love for God and bodybuilding had come to represent two dichotomies: the importance of spiritual health versus physical health. Was my physical (including mental health) just as important as my spiritual health? How does the Apostle John in 3 John 1:2 answer this question?

_____

_____

_____

_____

15. Read 2 Corinthians 10:3-5 to answer the following questions:

    a. How does Paul describe the weapons we fight resistance with?

    _____

    _____

    b. What word is equated with **addiction** in 2 Corinthians 10:3-5?

    _____

    c. What type of weapons has God provided us? Read each scripture reference and
       identify the weapon.

       Psalm 43:5 _____

       Proverbs 17:22 _____

       Mark 9:28-29 (KJV) _____

       Philippians 4:6_____

       Hebrews 4:12 _____

16. Read Psalm 63:1-8. Write down at least one imagery or word pertaining to each of the
    five senses.

    a. Taste-

    b. Sight-

    c. Hear-

    d. Touch-

    e. Smell-

17. Why should the desire for God become greater than our strongest craving?

    _____

    _____

    _____

18. Name the 8 foods in *The Ten Guiding Lights to Health and Wholeness* that tend to feed addiction.

_____

_____

19. According to Philippians 2:12-13, how is God working in us?

_____

_____

_____

20. Based on *The Ten Guiding Lights to Health and Wholeness,* list the four reasons the first commandment is important.

_____

_____

_____

_____

Application:
Preparation for your Journey

- Keep a food journal. Make copies of the chart in appendix A. Or you may use a digital app or an online program to keep a record.

- Limit your coffee intake to one cup per day. Coffee/ caffeine raises the metabolic rate and helps to mobilize fatty acids from the fat tissues. It can also enhance physical performance. However, caffeine is a stimulant and can be addictive once its stimulation wears off.
  Alternative: Drink green tea which is loaded with antioxidants. Green tea also lowers one's risk of cancer and has been shown to boost the metabolic rate, which increases fat burning in the short term although not all studies agree. Drink as many cups of tea as desired.

- Alcohol is a drug and, therefore, is best avoided, especially by individuals who cannot keep their drinking to a moderate.

- Chocolate, in particular milk chocolate, contains large amounts of saturated fat, caffeine, sugar and an array of sugary and fattening flavorings and fillings. Remove this food from your diet. However, an occasional dark chocolate is known to have some health benefits. Dark chocolate is high in flavanols – substances that help lower blood pressure and improve vascular function, improve cognitive function, and even provides UV protection for our skin! Dark chocolate has a higher proportion of flavanols than milk chocolate.

- Bread should be 100% whole grain. Remove all white breads and any bread that is not 100% whole grain.

- Instead of baked treats eat fruits. Avoid all desserts if one is trying to lose weight until one is able to balance one's intake with what one expends.

- Chips/pretzels should be removed.

- Fruity candy, mints, gum should be removed.

- About 75 percent of the world's population is genetically unable to properly digest milk and other dairy products because of a problem called lactose intolerance. Get calcium from dark green vegetables, almonds and other products such as almond milk. Dairy products, such as ice cream and cow's milk should be avoided. However, there are ice creams made from coconut milk that can be substituted if one desired a treat. (A treat is considered one day out of the week.)

Checking In:

Submit your food journal to your accountability partner. See appendix A.

Keep a record of your daily exercise. See Appendix C. Remember to walk as much as possible even if you are fit and healthy.

Reflection (in your journal):

Take time to reflect at the end of each week. Or if you feel compelled to write during the week, you may do so as well. What were the challenges you faced since beginning the journey? What were your successes or failures? Are you depending on God to help you rather than making changes within your own strength?

Notes:

1. Rex Russell, *What the Bible Says about Healthy Living: Three Biblical Principles That Will Change Your Diet and Improve Your Health* (Bloomington, Minnesota: Bethany House Publishers, 2006), 91.
2. William Struthers, *Wired for Intimacy: How Pornography Hijacks the Male Brain* (Downers Grove, IL: InterVarsity Press, 2009), 90, Kindle edition.
3. Myles Munroe, *Rediscovering the Kingdom: Ancient Hope for Our 21st Century World* (Shippensburg, PA: Destiny Image Publishers, 2004), 97.
4. Romans 12:1 (NIV).
5. Joan Chittister, *The Rule of Benedict: Insights for the Ages* (New York, NY: The Crossroad Publishing Company, 1992), 65.

Chapter 2

Do Not Idolize Your Body

"You must not make for yourself an idol of any kind or an image of anything in the heavens or on the earth or in the sea."

Goals:
Aim to exercise for at least 150 minutes each week
Develop a holistic attitude toward health and wellness
Understand the image Christ Jesus has restored me to
Understand how my health and wellness relate to God's kingdom message
Understand how the second commandment protects and restores my health and well being

Objectives:
Define shame
Recognize the importance of exercise
Exercise responsible food choices
Eat only foods that God has blessed
Evaluate my mental image of myself
Choose one of the following goals above to focus on for the week

Your goal for this week:

_____

_____

Today, we live in a world that places great emphasis on being healthy and fit. Though still trailing behind, the church is now becoming an active participant in doing its part in promoting a healthy lifestyle. However, we must be cautious that we do not follow the world's definition of health. The world says to be healthy, you have to look a certain way; it is all about the image. Though it is important to look healthy, it is not all about the image. If we are not careful, we will follow these image chasers, modeling ourselves after what the media portray as "healthy." Instead, we must first learn to see ourselves through the spiritual mirror— the Word of God.

1. Why is it important to address our body image within a God context?

_____

_____

Self-Idolization

Self-idolization was the result of Adam's and Eve's disobedience. In Genesis 3:1-8, Satan had promised Adam and Eve that if they ate from the tree of knowledge of good and evil, they would become like God. This desire to be like God was not the problem, for they were already god-like, being created in the image of God. Instead, Adam and Eve thought they could be like God without God. As a result, Adam's and Eve's vulnerability and inadequacy were exposed. In shame, they covered themselves with fig leaves and hid themselves. How could they be their true selves without God? Anything achieved outside of God was an illusion and was detrimental to their well-being and health. Thus, sickness, pain, hatred—shame was birth. Adam and Eve fell "short of God's glorious ideal."[1] Like them, we, too, have tried to create an image of how we think we should look, act and be. "This is the person we would like to be—a person of our own creation, the person we would create if we were God."[2] This gap between the person we would like to be and "the reality of what and who we are" is shame.[3]

Today, shame is the face behind many of our body-image issues. Many problems, "such as sexual and emotional abuse, drug and alcohol addiction, and eating disorders are shame-based and "treatment is often sabotaged or inadequate unless the shame core in these illnesses is worked through."[4]

2. How is shame defined in the above lines?

_____

_____

3. Why were Adam and Eve considered to be god-like?

_____

_____

4. What did they want?

_____

_____

5. According to Romans 3: 23, what was the result of pursuing this goal?

_____

_____

6. How have we tried to create an idol of ourselves?

_____

_____

7. Why is *shame* defined as the gap between the person we would like to be and the reality of who and what we are?

_____

_____

8. When we think about health and wellness, we all have an image in mind. What is that image you see? How do you see yourself? (Continue in your journal)

_____

_____

_____

Remembering Who We Really Are

The questions above are critical because they affect our well-being. The way we perceive ourselves determines how we feel. If we like the way we look, we feel good about ourselves. If we see ourselves as successful, then we may feel good about ourselves. But what happens if something changes? If we become less attractive due to a sickness or we lose our jobs? Then our self-esteem and self-worth are flushed down the toilet. Our self-worth cannot be based on what we accomplish or on our appearance. Nothing in this life is permanent. Our worth needs to be grounded on the essence or the make-up of our being, and that is spiritual. God is spirit, and we are created in His likeness.

If we are created in God's image, then we are also spiritual beings. According to the biblical narrative of Adam and Eve, we are like God in terms of attributes. We, too, possess the ability to create like our Creator. But through the Fall of humanity, we have lost or forgotten who we truly are as God's children. Instead, we have replaced our Creator with images of other human beings or things. Perhaps our graven image is to attain a particular physique. I know it was for me when I was competing in bodybuilding competitions. I remember battling, struggling—trying to find that space for God when all I could see was "I." I had become my own graven image. And in seeing only myself, I saw only my flaws and shortcomings. I was not big enough; I was too small to be a bodybuilder, I thought. This is what happens when we create an image of likeness that is not God. We become self-conscious, imprisoned by the image. We are not good enough. That thing or person becomes our master, and we become subservient to it because our emotions tell us: If our emotions are right and good, then they make us healthy. If they are toxic and wrong, then they make us sick eventually. Sometimes, we do not realize the damage they have done to us until we find ourselves stuck in the mud of addiction or some mental illness.

Self-acceptance

Our bodies are unashamedly marvelously wonderful creations. It does not matter what you or I think about our bodies. What matters is what God says about us.

13

9. Memorize and say **Psalm 139-13-18**. Be courageous and say these verses aloud in front of the mirror.

Self-acceptance is not idolatrous. It only becomes if the love for oneself becomes independent of and greater than God. However, we have to become aware of our natural tendency to attach to idols so that we can be intentional about attaching to God and his kingdom. This connection is not limited simply to the spiritual life but to all facets of life. Through God all life exists. He defines the ocean's shoreline. He establishes the water's boundaries.[5] Likewise, it is God who also establishes the boundaries of our body. If we jump from a building, we fall: it's called the law of gravity. If we plant a seed in the ground, a plant grows and bears fruit: It's called the law of sowing and reaping. If we sit most of the day and consume a high carbohydrate diet, we gain weight: It's called the law of cause and effect. Giving ourselves the right foods and proper physical, mental, and spiritual exercises are critical to our entire well-being. We cannot just feed ourselves spiritually, and ignorance of this fact is, perhaps, one of the reasons many Christians are dying from lifestyle diseases and going to heaven before their time.

10. Who defines the boundaries governing our bodies? What happens when we violate them?

_____

_____

_____

From the very beginning, God created human beings and provided for their bodies food from His garden that would nurture and energize them.

Food from God's Garden
Read Genesis 1:27-31.

11. What evidence in Scripture is there to support that Adam and Eve ate only plants?

_____

_____

_____

12. What type of food did God provide for the animals?

_____

_____

13. What is revealed about the food that was supposed to be eaten?

_____

_____

_____

Examples of Seed-Bearing Plants	
Whole grains	Whole oats, brown rice, millet, barley, corn on the cob, whole rye, quinoa
Dried beans	Lentils, garbanzo beans, split peas, kidney beans, pinto beans, navy beans, black or yellow soybeans, black-eyed peas, great northern beans
Vegetables	Leafy greens (spinach, collard greens, turnip greens), root vegetables (sweet potato, potato, yucca), sea vegetable (seaweed)
Fruit	Berries, apples, pears, melons, cantaloupe, peaches
Nuts/seeds	Almonds, walnuts, pecans, cashew, sesame, sunflower, pumpkin, flax, linseed

Within a seed, God planted life. We are to eat life to beget life. As a result, these plants are considered **living**. How many of us did the experiment in elementary school where we placed a bean in a tissue and put it in a jar? We kept it moist with water. In a few days, we noticed it sprout. That seed has **life** in it. If we took the stalks of some green plants and put them in water, they too will begin to grow. Root vegetables will grow too if we replant them. What happens when we leave an uncooked potato for too long? We begin to see a stem appearing. These foods are still living, whereas processed foods such as white bread and pasta, canned foods, sugary boxed cereals, frozen fish sticks and dinners, packaged cakes and cookies, and processed meats (hot dogs, sausage, lunch meats) are **dead.** They have been chemically altered by human beings. On the other hand, God created vegetables, fruits, and nuts with His very hands to give us life. They contain nutrients to nourish us and healing properties to heal us. These foods should also be prepared in such a way as to protect the nutrients in them. They should never be fried. Steaming, sautéing, boiling, pressure cooking, and baking are some ways to preserve the nutrients.

Because these living foods or whole foods are in their natural state rather than processed, they help to keep us balanced by keeping our blood sugar levels stable.

We should plan our meals around 3 food categories: carbohydrates, proteins, and fats. The seed-bearing plants are going to be called our preferred or good carbohydrates in this study.

Carbohydrates, which are sugar and starches, are the body's preferred fuel. The body will seek for this type of fuel first before it goes to the next energy source—fat. Our complex carbohydrates are our whole grains and starchy vegetables, such as quinoa and sweet potato. The amount of carbohydrates we consume is going to depend on our activity level.

For example, when training as a body builder, my diet was made up of 60% carbohydrate. I needed the energy to lift as heavy as possible. However, once competition season began, my carbohydrates were reduced significantly, making it very challenging to train at optimum level but needed in order to lose the fat. I had to make another dietary adjustment when I stopped competing. Because I was not training as a body builder any longer, I had to reduce my carbohydrate again. I no longer needed that amount of fuel to work out. Any excess calories that were not used would be stored as fat, and I knew this, so I gradually reduced my *desire* for a predominantly carbohydrate diet.

Many of us, consume too many carbohydrates. As a result, we are storing excess fat. Carbohydrate stimulates insulin, a hormone, and an excess amount of insulin makes us fat and keeps us fat. If we are athletes, we would need more carbohydrate than individuals who have a sit-down job. But, most of us are not athletes. Therefore, we need to be careful about the type and the amount of carbohydrates we consume.

Vegetables, such as leafy greens, are also carbohydrates, known as fibrous carbohydrates. Although they are a part of the carbohydrate family, these types of vegetables do not impact our blood sugar level in the way complex carbohydrates do. Because fiber has very little impact on the blood sugar level, insulin production is controlled. Most of our carbohydrates should, therefore, come from fibrous carbohydrates—vegetables.

God, the Master Gardener and Creator, certainly knew what He was doing when He provided these foods for Adam and Eve. He designed their bodies—our bodies—to function optimally on vegetables.

Keeping the Garden Fit
Physiologically, food was necessary for Adam and Eve's bodies, providing energy for them to carry out their responsibilities to take care of the garden and to protect it. Exercise would naturally be a part of their lives, and food would be used to sustain them to fulfill God's work—the care of His garden.

   14. Circle the ACTION words in the scripture below:

"The Lord God put the man in the Garden of Eden to care for it and work it" (Gen 2:15).

Read the following verses:

Before Disobedience

Genesis 2:15

The LORD God placed the man in the Garden of Eden to tend and watch over it.

After Disobedience

Genesis 3: 17-19

To Adam he said, "Because you listened to your wife and ate fruit from the tree about which I commanded you, 'You must not eat from it,'

> "Cursed is the ground because of you;
> through painful toil you will eat food from it
> all the days of your life.
> It will produce thorns and thistles for you,
> and you will eat the plants of the field.
> By the sweat of your brow
> you will eat your food
> until you return to the ground,
> since from it you were taken;
> for dust you are
> and to dust you will return." (NIV)

15. How does Adam and Eve's punishment differ before and after the great Fall?

_____

_____

_____

_____

_____

I smile when I hear people, in particular women, say they dislike sweating. Sweating is healthy and necessary, and it also signifies our human nature to struggle. In Genesis 3:19, God condemns Adam and Eve to a life of hardship: "By the sweat of your brow will you have food to eat until you return to the ground from which you were made." The element of resistance is embedded in life. Some say life is wounded; others say it is what it is. We have to accept the hard work that now comes with maintaining our body, mind and spirit. God is not going to zap us with what we can do for ourselves, no matter how much we believe in the supernatural.

Furthermore, just to show how merciful God is, He gave us the ability to perspire in order to remove waste products and to cool our body when it reaches a certain temperature. So the ability to perspire is also a gift. Here is another perceptual shift. Some of us may dislike exercise but again God shows us His incredible mercy by allowing us to experience wonderful endorphins— "the feel good hormones"—as a result of disciplining our bodies. In addition, exercise enables us to stay healthy by controlling weight, warding off diseases, reducing stress, improving self-confidence, preventing cognitive decline, alleviating anxiety, helping with addiction, promoting better sleep, improving one's sex life, boosting energy and creativity, and creating mental space to think, reflect, meditate and to hear God.

16. Not all of us enjoy exercising. Some of us see exercise as a form of punishment, pain or even a curse. What are two mental shifts we can make to change this attitude towards exercise? How does God show his loving kindness towards us despite The Fall of humankind?

_____

_____

_____

_____

17. During the Middle Ages, the church recognized seven sins as fatal to spiritual growth. They were pride, covetousness, lust, anger, gluttony, envy, and sloth. Two of these are mentioned in chapter one of *The Ten Guiding Lights to Health and Wholeness*.

Name two that speak to you personally. Why have you chosen these two?

_____

_____

_____

_____

18. Read Proverbs 6:6 and 20:4 and Ecclesiastes 10:18. What does the Bible say about slothfulness?

_____

_____

_____

_____

19. How does the second command protect your health and well-being?

_____

_____

Application:

Beginning Your Journey

- Walk every day—all the days of your life. No matter your fitness level, look for the opportunity to get a few extra steps in your day.

- If *exercising*, walk vigorously, swinging arms for at least 30 minutes 5 days a week. Your breathing should change but you should be able to speak.

- Include weights as you walk or include weight training.

- If you have a sit-down job, make it your goal to get up every 1-2 hours. Take a 5-20-minute break to walk or stretch.

Checking In:

Submit your food journal to your accountability partner. See appendix A.

Keep a record of your daily exercise. See appendix C. Remember to walk as much as possible even if you are fit and healthy.

Reflection (in your journal):

How do you see yourself physically and mentally? Do not talk about how you should see yourself. Why do you see yourself in this way?

"Walking is a man's best medicine." — Hippocrates

Notes:

1. Romans 3:23 (TLB).
2. David Benner, *The Gift of Being Yourself: The Sacred Call to Self-Discovery* (Downer Grove, IL: InterVarsity Press, 2004), 80, Kindle edition.
3. David F. Allen, *Shame: The Human Nemesis*, (Nassau, Bahamas: Eleuthera Publications, 2010), 17.
4. Allen, *Shame: The Human Nemesis*, 17.
5. Proverbs 8:29.

Chapter 3

Do Not Devalue God's Name

"You must not use the name of the Lord your God thoughtlessly; the Lord will punish anyone who misuses his name."

Goals:
Aim to exercise for at least 150 minutes each week
Develop a holistic attitude toward health and wellness
Understand how I can misrepresent God's name
Understand how the third commandment calls our attention to the name we represent

Objectives:
Identify foods God forbids to be eaten
Exercise responsible food choices
Eat only foods that God has blessed
Choose one of the following goals above to focus on for the week

Your goal for this week:

_____

_____

A name has power; it has value. To name a thing is to acknowledge its existence separate from all other things that exist. To name means to pay attention—to identify. Perhaps, this ability to name explains why the ancient Hebrews had numerous names for God. These names revealed or called attention to God's character and presence. Such was the case regarding the name Yahweh — "I am who I am."[1] In other words, Yahweh means "to be." This name is often referred to as the unutterable name of God that is so holy it cannot be spoken. As a result, various substitutes, such as Jehovah, Adonai, Hashem, El Shaddai, are used. This custom is to avoid breaking the third commandment, which forbids the thoughtless use of the name of the Lord. The prohibition quite naturally included the use of profanity or any false representation of God. It also underscores the fact that God wants to engage us fully—body, mind and spirit. He wants us to be aware and mindful of the way we use His name, which reflects His power and glory. He is the essence of our being—the source of all life.

This respect for God's name was also conferred on earthly kings who were recognized as God's representatives on earth. From ancient times, when the king's name was used on a document it could not be revoked; it was law. An example of this power is seen in the story of Esther. When King Ahasuerus sent out an order to exterminate the Jews, the order read:

> "Now go ahead and send a message to the Jews in the king's name, telling them whatever you want, and seal it with the king's signet ring. But remember that whatever has already been written in the king's name and sealed with his signet ring can never be revoked."[2]

1. What did the king's name represent?

_____

_____

2. What was the consequence if the king's name was falsely represented?

_____

_____

The king's name represented the king himself. Any misuse or misrepresentation of his name was punishable by death. Hence, this third commandment reflects the reverence and honor given to the King of all kings. Normally, we recognize the misuse of God's name when it is associated with profanity or used in oath taking. However, a closer look, we can also misrepresent God's name through our lifestyle—the way we live. The Israelites' lifestyle branded them as God's people. Whatever they did was a replication of their honor to God. This devotion to God was also exemplified in the story of Daniel and his three friends—Hananiah, Mishael, and Azariah, all of whose names were later changed to Belteshazzar, Shadrach, Meshach, and Abednego when Jerusalem was captured by King Nebuchadnezzar of Babylon.

King Nebuchadnezzar wanted several of the captured Israelites to become members of the royal court. Daniel and three of his friends were amongst the men chosen. While in the King's service, Daniel and his comrades chose not to eat the King's food. Clarke's (1834/2011) commentary said there were three reasons Daniel probably chose not to eat the Kings food:[3]

- Because they ate unclean beasts which were forbidden by Jewish law.
- Because they ate, as did the heathens in general, beasts which had been strangled or not properly blooded.
- Because the animals that were eaten were first offered as victims to their gods.

Quite simply, the food was not kosher.

3. Read Daniel chapter 1. What did Daniel request from the king's guard?

_____

_____

4. How long would this test last?

_____

5. Describe the appearance of Daniel and his friends after this period of time.

_____

_____

_____

6. How did Daniel honor the name of God?

_____

_____

7. What blessing did Daniel gain for honoring what was holy to God?

_____

_____

_____

8. How can we apply this lesson to our own lives?

_____

_____

_____

Although the act of honoring kosher for these ancient Hebrews was primarily for spiritual reasons, we can also see today the health benefits of limiting our animal intake and consuming more plants as was intended.

It appears that there was a change after the great Deluge when everything was destroyed, including the vegetation, that an animal-based diet required special instructions. In the ark with Noah and his family were the animals. In Deuteronomy 14:3-21, God gave these guidelines regarding the meat to be consumed:

Mammals that *made* the team and may be eaten
These animals have split hooves with even number of toes and they chew their cud.

9. Give 4 examples of these animals.

_____

Mammals that *did not* make the team and are not to be eaten

Complete the following sentences with the correct animal.

10. Although the _____ has a split hoof, it does not chew its cud. The _____ has only one toe but does not have a split hoof. The _____ and the _____ do not have hooves.

According to *Encyclopedia of Foods and Their Healing Power*, there are two possible reasons the animals with split hooves and who chew their cuds would be considered fit for human consumption:

(i) These animals eat plants and so they are called herbivores. Animals that eat plants tend to carry less toxic residue and contaminants because they are on a lower position on the food chain. Hence, if one is to eat meat, animals raised on grass would be preferred to animals on commercial feed.

(ii) In addition, these animals, which are plant eaters, contain "a complex gastric system consisting of four sacs in which everything is fermented and chemically disinfected to some degree before it passes to the intestine and into the bloodstream."[4]

11. Why is it better to eat animals that eat plants?

_____

_____

_____

Aquatic animals not to be eaten

Fish that do not have fins and scales are not to be consumed.

12. Give 4 examples of these fishes.

_____

These sea creatures have a high urea content, which makes them toxic. In addition, these fish are carnivores, which mean they eat other animals. As a result, they contain "the highest concentrates of mercury and other toxins."[5]

Shellfish are not recommended to be eaten because of what they consume and where they live. These aquatic animals act like sea vultures. They feed on dead and decaying animals, moving across the ocean floor as they cleanse the sea from remains and organic waste. As a result, these sea creatures "accumulate the most contaminants and toxins"[6] and "anyone eating shellfish is taking in seawater concentrated with all of its pollutants."[7]

13. What are "sea vultures?" Give an example.

_____

_____

Fowls not to be eaten

14. Give two examples of birds that are not to be consumed.

_____

Reptiles

15. What reptiles are allowed to be eaten?

_____

The Meat Dilemma

Whether to eat meat has always been a prickly subject. But, as the statistics pile in, more and more data are showing that folks who eat a high-meat diet have an increased risk of cardiac, cardiovascular, and rheumatic-related diseases. Research also shows that a high animal protein diet raises the risk of various cancers.[8]

Unfortunately, the consumption of vegetables and fruits and daily prayers has been allocated to a fast called the Daniel Fast. Many Christians have participated in this fast. The benefits of this way of eating are numerous: weight loss and healings from diseases such as diabetes, cancer, and allergies. Some addictions are even broken as the body detoxifies itself. Yet, despite the benefits of these foods, many Christians discontinue a diet high in these types of fibrous carbohydrates and resort to old ways of eating, such as a diet high in meat, once the fast has ended. Eating a diet high in vegetables and fruits should not be called a fast when it was a prescribed diet from the very beginning.

Many of us would say, "But, I do eat fruits and vegetables." The question, then, is do you eat enough of them? What is the main food on your plate? Is your meal planned around meat or vegetables? Is meat the main dish on your plate?

16. Give three (3) reasons why vegetables and fruits should be the staple foods in our diet??

_____

_____

_____

_____

_____

17. Give three (3) reasons why we should be cautious about our meat intake.

_____

_____

_____

18. During this week, note how many vegetables and fruits and meat you consume (copy chart from Appendix B). Keep a record of your intake in your food journal. Do you eat vegetables with each meal? Can you increase your vegetables, in particular the green vegetables, and lessen your meat consumption?

Scripture says, "God never changes his mind about the people he calls and the things he gives them."[9] It is noteworthy to study the dietary guidelines given by God. If it is important to God, then it should be important to us. Yes, God cares about what we eat or put in the body, for He expects us to honor Him with our bodies too! He has given us the power to choose and the ability to exercise self-control. We must show discipline even at the table not just in spiritual matters as we so often think. We may not like vegetables, but it is important to learn to eat them. We may not be used to having vegetables as the main food item on our plates, but if they make us healthier, is it not better? We may not like protein, but if it is the essential nutrient to our bodies, we need to incorporate it. When we were children, our parents made us eat our vegetables (or at least some of us) and made us go to bed on time. Now that we are adults, we need to train ourselves to eat our vegetables and go to bed on time.

19. How does the third commandment protect your health and well-being?

_____

_____

Application:

Being Mindful on your Journey

- Keep a record of the amount of vegetables, fruits and meat you consume in your food journal. Copy the chart from Appendix B.

- Eat your fruits preferably in the morning in order to use their energy throughout the day.

- Eat fruits with their skin in order to benefit from the fiber, which also helps in keeping the blood sugar level stable.

- Beginning this week, your vegetables should make up the main food on your plate.

See the diagram below:

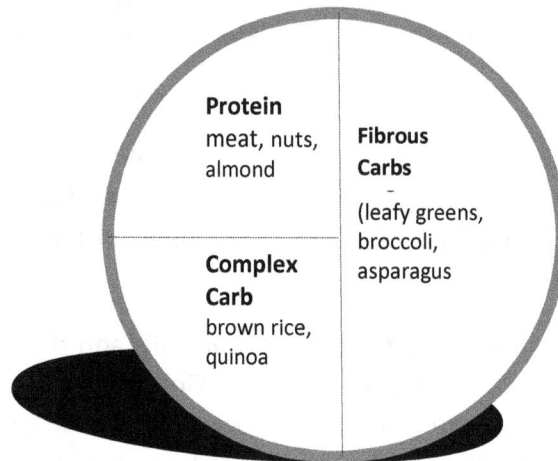

Protein
meat, nuts, almond

Fibrous Carbs - (leafy greens, broccoli, asparagus

Complex Carb
brown rice, quinoa

You should have more fibrous vegetables such as leafy greens, broccoli, and asparagus than the complex carbohydrates such as brown rice, sweet potato, or quinoa.

- EXPAND YOUR TERRITORY: Buy a fruit you have never tasted. Describe its taste, texture, look and smell, and even sound when you eat it.

- EXPAND YOUR TERRITORY: Buy a vegetable you have never tasted. Describe its taste, texture, look and smell, and even sound when you eat it.

- EXPAND YOUR TERRITORY: Buy a whole grain you have never tasted. Describe its taste, texture, look and smell, and even sound when you eat it.

☑ Checking In:

Submit your food journal to your accountability partner. See appendix B.

Keep a record of your daily exercise. See appendix C. Remember to walk as much as possible even if you are fit and healthy.

Reflection (in your journal):

Are you honoring God with your body? How have you not honored him with your body? How have you honored him with your body? Your examples do not have to be related to food.

Notes:

1. Exodus 3:14.
2. Esther 8:8.
3. Adam Clarke. "Commentary on Daniel 1:8. *The Adam Clarke Commentary.* http://www.studylight.org/commentaries/acc/daniel-1.html. 1832.
4. George D. Pamplona-Roger. *Encyclopedia of Foods and Their Healing Power*, s.v. "Fish and Shellfish." Vol. 1, 297. Madrid: Editorial Safeliz.
5. Pamplona-Roger, 245.
6. Pamplona-Roger, 252.
7. Pamplona-Roger, 258.
8. Pamplona-Roger. *Encyclopedia of Foods and Their Healing Power*, s.v. "Meat." 263.
9. Romans 11:29.

Chapter 4

Live a Balanced Life

"Remember to observe the Sabbath day by keeping it holy."

Goals:

Recognize the different types of rest

Understand the significance of the Sabbath

Aim to exercise for at least 150 minutes each week

Develop a holistic attitude toward health and wellness

Learn how to relax the body naturally to aid in spiritual growth

Realize the importance of rest for health, healing and productivity

Understand how the forth commandment protects and restores our health and well being

Objectives:

Sleep 6-8 hours

Practice relaxing the body

Honor the Sabbath as a time of rest

Meditate on a scripture pertaining to peace

Recognize the impact of sleep deprivation

Explain why rest is important to the body physically, emotionally, mentally and spiritually

Choose one of the following goals above to focus on for the week

Your goal for this week:

_____

_____

God instructs us to "[w]ork and get everything done during six days each week" and "the seventh day is a day of rest to honor" Him.[1]

For many, the Sabbath is actually Sunday. This change was officially made by Roman Emperor Constantine on March 7, 321. Many Christians, dating back to the time of Ignatius of Antioch (c.115), the third bishop of Antioch, believed that the Sabbath should be about spiritual matters only. The Sabbath was, indeed, also spiritual, for Christ himself is declared to be *The Sabbath* where we would find rest also for our souls.[2]

The Sabbath is also recognized as a time for the contemplation of nature and the celebration of life—God's work of art! Upon completion of creation, God rested on the seventh day, which is called the Sabbath and in Hebrew *Shabbat*. The word Sabbath or *Shabbat* is a period of cessation and rest. By naming a day Sabbath, God calls our attention to the body's need for relaxation and rest, which is also a part of His creation.

1. Write out the following scriptures and identify the aspect of the Sabbath that each of the scriptures refer to.

   (i) Exodus 20:9-10a.

   _____

   _____

   _____

   (ii) Exodus 20:11.

   _____

   _____

   _____

   (iii) Matthew 11:28.

   _____

   _____

   _____

Understanding the need for rest was one of the most important and difficult lessons for me to learn. This wake-up call occurred a few years ago. I was involved in an accident. I had gotten very little sleep for several nights. I had no idea that I had crossed a red light. I hit a car head on and then another. Thankfully, no one was hurt, and I walked away with only a scratch—not even a delayed muscle ache or soreness, which I owe to God and my fitness level at the time. My car, however, was a total write-off, but I realized that God spared my life from a situation I had created. I was abusing my body. I did not feel I needed six or seven hours of sleep. I thought three to four hours of sleep and sometimes less were sufficient. Obviously, my body felt otherwise, for I had fallen asleep in broad daylight. I had put myself in danger. If an alcoholic and I had anything in common, it would be our addictions. Though I identified my addiction as "workaholism," my cognitive impairment and motor performance were the same as "a legally prescribed level of alcohol intoxication."[3] In other words, I might as well had been drunk.

2. Why is a sleep deprived person like a legally drunk individual?

_____

_____

Sleep deprivation affects us physically, mentally and spiritually.

God has gifted each of us with a purpose. Whether we are aware of this purpose or not, Satan's plan will always be to prevent us from fulfilling what God has called us to do. However, we cannot always throw a "Flip Wilson" line—"the devil made me to do it." The responsibility lies on us to discipline ourselves. Making sure we receive sufficient sleep is one of those disciplines. As believers, we are not physically immune to the effects of sleep deprivation.

Sleep loss leads to the various problems:[4]

- impaired glucose tolerance (a pre-diabetic state; glucose above normal levels)
- decreased insulin sensitivity (the body requires more insulin, a hormone, to reduce blood sugar)
- increased evening concentrations of cortisol (a stress hormone that encourages fat storage)
- increased levels of ghrelin (a hormone that increases hunger)
- decreased levels of leptin (a hormone that helps us to feel full after eating)
- increased appetite
- increased sedentary behavior because of a lack of energy
- increased risk of obesity

All of these factors contribute to weight gain. When we are sleep-deprived, the hormone ghrelin increases, which stimulates hunger and the appetite for certain foods (particularly high in calorie). Leptin is a protein hormone that sends a signal to the brain to alert the body that it is full or has reached a point of satiety. When the body has not received adequate rest, that hormone is reduced, resulting in overeating since the body is less aware when it is full. When this happens, the body secretes insulin to manage the glucose or sugar levels in the blood. Insulin, a hormone, carries the glucose and stores it in the liver, muscles and cells as glycogen—stored energy. Any excess is stored as fat. As long as there are high levels of insulin, the body will not use its stored fat as energy. Too much glucose in the blood can result in impaired glucose tolerance and can also lead to reduced insulin sensitivity where the body requires more insulin to manage the high levels of sugar in the blood.

When these physiological conditions lead to obesity, a host of other medical problems develop:

- hypertension
- diabetes mellitus
- elevated cholesterol
- coronary heart disease

- renal disease (kidney failure)
- cerebrovascular accident (stroke)
- pulmonary complications
- arthritis
- cancer

Sleep loss affects the body's ability to balance, restore, and heal itself the way God designed it. Sleep deprivation is, in essence, a form of slow death.

In Acts 20, while sitting in an open window and listening to one of Paul's long sermons that lasted until midnight, a young man named Eutychus goes to sleep, falls from the third floor and dies. Thankfully, Paul miraculously heals the young man and brings him back to life. Many times, we fill our lives up with activities at work, church and home. Though these are all good places to work or serve in, we neglect the care of our bodies if we are not receiving sufficient hours of sleep. Though God heals and restores as He has shown us, it is our responsibility to take care of the body and not to take advantage of His grace and mercy. If God had to rest, what about us? We become easy targets for the enemy when we are physically exhausted. Just as Eutychus fell asleep and fell out of the window, so Satan seeks to destroy us in any way possible, especially when we are physically weary and weak.

3. Don't test God.

Read 1 Corinthians 10:9. How did the people test God?

_____

_____

When we purposely do not rest our bodies, we can inflict harm on ourselves. How can this action be seen as testing God?

_____

_____

4. Don't be a target for the enemy.

Read 1 Peter 5:8. How does the scripture instruct us to behave?

_____

_____

How can this instruction relate to a lack of sleep?

_____

_____

5. Realize your importance to God's Plan even if it is not clear to you yet.

Read John 10:10. What does the scripture warn us?

_____

_____

How can this warning relate to sleep deprivation?

_____

_____

6. Stay mentally focused.

Read Proverbs 4:20-27. What advice does the parent give to his son that will call for him being and staying mentally alert?

_____

_____

_____

_____

The brain needs sleep and rest. A research study by University of California at Berkeley and Harvard Medical School purports that sleep deprivation boosts "the part of the brain most closely connected to depression, anxiety and other psychiatric disorders."[5] This information has significant implications, then, for keeping and maintaining healthy emotions. It suggests that during sleep our emotions and feelings are restored to a balanced state. If our body is the sanctuary of the Holy Spirit, then we need to become familiar with its functionality as much as possible, because God will use our body, including its brain, to accomplish his kingdom-agenda. God requires us to "be alert and of sober mind."[6] He is constantly speaking to us; it is up to us to be aware.

In this chapter on rest, we introduced some technical terms that may be new to some. So let's review:

7. When the body is sleep deprived, leptin is reduced, resulting in _____.

8. When there is an increase of sugar in the blood, the body secretes _____ to manage it.

9. If hormone _____ increases, one feels hungry.

10. Stress increases the hormone _____, which leads to _____.

11. Match the word on the right with the correct definition.

1._____ Leptin		a. the name for sugar in the blood
2._____ Ghrelin		b. hormone that tells the body it is full or satisfied
3._____ Insulin		c. a stress hormone that encourages fat storage
4._____ Glucose		d. insufficient sleep
5._____ Glycogen		e. hormone for managing blood sugar level
6._____ Sleep Deprivation		f. hormone for stimulating hunger and appetite
7._____ Cortisol		g. energy stored in the liver, muscles and cells

Rest and relaxation are both important to our body, mind and spirit. In order to cultivate a quiet heart, we have to learn to relax the body. Diaphragm breathing, which singers and actors practice, for example, can be used to help the body to relax. Newberg et al. recommend focusing on words such as "love" and "peace": "If you intensely focus on a word like "peace" or "love," the emotional centers in the brain calm down. The outside world hasn't changed at all, but you will still feel more safe and secure."[7]

There is a beautiful scripture in Isaiah 26:3 that supports this feeling of comfort and safety. The word peace comes from the Hebrew word "shalom" meaning completeness, soundness, welfare, and peace:[8]

> "You will keep in perfect peace those whose minds are steadfast, because they trust in you."

Allow yourself to not only take in the word "peace" but also the revelation that this scripture points to the God of peace—Jehovah Shalom. Take a few minutes to breathe in this scripture and exhale any worries, doubts, confusion or restless thoughts.

1. Begin by sitting upright in a chair.
2. Relax your body by allowing yourself to go limp.
3. Breathe deeply, inhaling through your nose and exhaling through your mouth.
4. Allow each word of the scripture to soak into your being.
5. Trust God with your anxious thoughts.
6. Offer them to Him because He cares about you.
7. As you breathe in his peace, exhale and let go off your concerns.
8. Meditate on the scripture as needed to cultivate God's peace.

12. How does the forth commandment protect your health and well-being?

_____

_____

Application:

Rest for Your Journey

- **Before retiring for bed, read and meditate on the verses from Proverbs 3:21-26 (MSG):** Dear friend, guard Clear Thinking and Common Sense with your life; don't for a minute lose sight of them. They'll keep your soul alive and well, they'll keep you fit and attractive. You'll travel safely, you'll neither tire nor trip. You'll take afternoon naps without a worry, you'll enjoy a good night's sleep. No need to panic over alarms or surprises, or predictions that doomsday's just around the corner, because God will be right there with you; he'll keep you safe and sound.

- **Sabbath Walk**
  Take a nature walk or spend a few minutes outdoors. Notice your environment as if you are seeing it for the first time. Write a poem or short description of your observation in your journal.

- Do you have a bedtime ritual? Share it with the group.

  If you do not have bedtime ritual, you can use Isaiah 26:3 as a scripture to meditate on before retiring. Carry out the act of sitting still and breathing deeply. See yourself handing over to God your agenda, cares or worries. Allow him to be the one who stays up and takes care of them while you sleep.

```
┌ ─ ─ ─ ─ ─ ─ ─ ─ ─ ─ ─ ─ ─ ─ ─ ─ ─ ─ ─ ─ ─ ─ ─ ─ ─ ─ ─ ─ ┐
```
Checking In:

Submit your food journal to your accountability partner. See appendix B.

Keep a record of your daily exercise. See appendix C. Remember to walk as much as possible even if you are fit and healthy.

Reflection (in your journal):

What's keeping you up? Think of a time you could not sleep. Describe what happened and what kept you up.
```
└ ─ ─ ─ ─ ─ ─ ─ ─ ─ ─ ─ ─ ─ ─ ─ ─ ─ ─ ─ ─ ─ ─ ─ ─ ─ ─ ─ ─ ┘
```

Notes:

1. Exodus 20:9-11 (NCV).
2. Matthew 12:8; Matthew 11:29
3. M. Williamson. "Moderate sleep deprivation produces impairments in cognitive and motor performance equivalent to legally prescribed levels of alcohol intoxication." *Occupational and Environmental Medicine*, 57, no.10 (June 2000): 649–655, accessed March 3, 2016. http://oem.bmj.com/content/57/10/649.short.
4. Guglielmo Beccuti. "Sleep and Obesity," *Clinical Nutrition and Metabolic Care*, 14, no. 4 (July 2011): 402-412, accessed March 29, (cited in abstract). doi: 10.1097/MCO.0b013e3283479109.
5. Yasmin Anwar. "Sleep Loss Linked to Psychiatric Disorders." *UC Berkeley News*, accessed March 29, 2016, (cited in press release). http://www.berkeley.edu/news/media/releases/2007/10/22_sleeploss.shtml.
6. 1 Peter 5:8 (NIV).
7. Andrew Newberg et al, *Words Can Change Your Brain: 12 Conversational Strategies to Build Trust, Resolve Conflict and Increase Intimacy* (New York, N.Y.: Penguin Group, 2012), 27.
8. *Lexicon-Concordance Online Bible*, s.v. "shalom." http://lexiconcordance.com/hebrew/7965.html.

Chapter 5

Cultivate Your Roots and You Will Grow

"Honor your father and mother. Then you will live a long, full life in the land the Lord your God is giving you."

Goals:
Understand aging as a gift of God
Improve our lives for the purpose of longevity
Understand the benefits of resistance training
Aim to exercise for at least 150 minutes each week
Develop a holistic attitude toward health and wellness
Improve upon the relationships in our lives for the purpose of our well-being
Understand how the fifth commandment protects and restores our health and well being

Objectives:
Eat foods with antioxidants
Prepare for a healthy, long life on earth
Capture a vision of how you want to age
Add resistance training in your workout
Choose one of the following goals above to focus on for the week

Your goal for this week:

_____

_____

Parents are not perfect. Yes, all parents have made mistakes, and some of these mistakes have affected their children's health and well-being. Yet, the Holy Scriptures give us a command to honor our parents—to esteem them. This commandment is a difficult pill to swallow when a parent becomes a child's enemy. I am sure God knew the mark of imperfection that would haunt all parents, so why would God emphasize that such high respect be given to parents? In addition, why would He tie this respect to longevity? God "enjoins us to honor our parents, not only for their sake, but for His. Honor shown to them is shown to God, for it acknowledges His claim as well"—as Father.[1]

Parents are the portals into this world. They are the portal of life that God has designed to bring us here. In other words, our parents are surrogates, and we are God's children. We attach to our earthly parents as children, for they become responsible for our health and well-being.

Therefore all relationships are birthed out of our parental connection. They become the "thread on which our own lives are strung."[2] How we relate to ourselves and how we relate to others are deeply affected by our relationships with our parents. Curt Thompson in *Anatomy of the Soul* describes this "physical universe through the birth canal" as the "portal of attachment."[3] Our relationships become contingent on how we relate to our caregivers. Our formative years become very critical in establishing our emotional and mental health. Many experts believe "the parent-child relationship could provide a "secure base" from which children could explore the world around them with confidence and security. These children could then develop emotional elasticity in the face of stress, build healthy relationships with peers and establish a sense of emotional equilibrium within their own minds."[4] Basically, if we are securely rooted in childhood, then we would have the stable ground to stand upon and to take on the world with confidence. Unfortunately, all of us have been insecurely attached—some more so than others.

Surrendering to God's Love

Paul, in encouraging the church in Ephesus, prayed that they would be deeply rooted and securely grounded in God's love.[5] Another word for "rooted" and "grounded" is "attached." This attachment is similar to the way tree roots behave in holding soil together. Without the roots the soil would fall away. Quite similarly, it is God's love that is supposed to hold us together. However, we have chosen to attach ourselves to the lesser things in life. We have attached ourselves to food to make us feel better when we need to be comforted. We have attached ourselves to drugs when we need something to uplift us or numb us so we do not feel the pain. We have attached ourselves to work to give us value. We have attached ourselves to our children to give us a sense of purpose. We have attached ourselves to relationships to make us feel loved. We have attached ourselves to our intellect so that we feel esteemed or significant. We have attached ourselves to self to make us feel in control. We can go on and on, naming all the things we attach ourselves to, and each one would be labeled an illusion.

The only true and permanent attachment is God. All the others are temporal and a shadow of the real. For example, eating a bowl of ice cream every night may result in happiness at the time of consumption but eventually it will certainly wreak havoc on the body. What about the pleasure of inactivity—watching television every night or spending hours on the computer or at work? What about the satisfaction from that cigarette or "joint" that alleviates the stress or provides some comfort? These indulgences may seem harmless, but they have the power to sabotage our physical and spiritual health and well-being. These objects, experiences, even people lead us to believe that the pleasure we derive from them would not be ours without their existence.[6] In other words, we give them ultimate value that we should give only to God. God is the one who satisfies our soul, which is really where our deep hunger and drive originate.

When we re-attach to God's love, it secures us; it roots us. The insecurities in life can uproot us, but an understanding of and complete surrender to God's love secures us. Surrendering to God's love grounds, sustains, nourishes, reassures, and completes us. In God's love we are good enough. Outside of God's love, we are continually searching, looking as if for the next "high" or the next big thing to make us feel significant or esteemed. His love has the power to heal in places no surgeon's scalpel can reach, to renew brain cells so that we remember events differently in the context of a God who sets free, who resurrects what was dead, and who gives purpose for living again. In God's love, we are finally safe and secure where even death cannot touch us. Paul asks what can separate us from the love of God? The answer, he says, is NOTHING.[7]

Growing in love rather than in fear is learning to live again. It means putting away some childish things, as Paul too had to do: "When I was a child, I spoke and thought and reasoned as a child. But when I grew up, I put away childish things."[8] Thompson explains that the "way people learn to manage emotional states as children will follow them into their adult friendships, marriages, and work relationships." But this state is not permanent; it can "change at any age [from insecure to secure or vice versa]."[9]

What are some childish things we may still practice? Let's take a look at some of them.

Parent-Pleasing to People-Pleasing
Read 2 Kings 14:1-7 and 2 Kings 15:1-6.

1. What did Amaziah and Azariah do to please the people? Why was it wrong to be a people pleaser?

_____

_____

Einstein's Definition of Insanity

Some diseases are also cyclic and have been passed down through generational lines in the manner in which we cook. Some of these cooking methods, which were once less harmful for a generation that walked and rode bicycles often, are deadly for our sedentary lifestyle. Is it any surprise, then, that certain cultures are predisposed to certain types of diseases such as hypertension or obesity? Einstein defines insanity as doing the same thing over and over again but expecting different results. Many times, we cook the way our mama cooked, and our mama cooked the way her mama cooked. I am not bad mouthing anybody's mama. The fact is cultural traditions may be hard to break at times, but we have to seek truth and follow truth. Now is the time to unlearn them and do things differently.

2. Think of some dishes you prepare. What are some recipes or cooking methods that have been passed down and may not be considered healthy?

_____

_____

_____

_____

The Game "Mama Said"

As kids, our parents told us to eat our vegetables. Some of us did; some of us did not. Now, as adults, generally, we still do not eat the amount of vegetables we should. A plant-based diet keeps us healthy and wards off diseases. Yet many people continue to eat a meat-based diet. Kara Davis, MD, author of *Spiritual Secrets to Weight Loss*, argues that "we don't need a 'diet' that adjusts our menu for a week or two; we need a 'diet' that will permanently change our attitude about food, our lifestyles, and the way we treat God's living temple. Our attitude must reflect a spirit of sacrificial love, which makes us willing to give up a few things we enjoy for the greater purpose of good health."[10]

3. Since starting this study, what sacrifice have you made for the betterment of your health?

_____

_____

The Peter Pan Syndrome

In general, we dread "the advance of old age. . . . One need only notice the ads in the magazines or the actors in the movies to realize that youth is our god; being young is divine. We spend more time concealing the 'disease' of age than healing diseases itself."[11] Growing old can be a fearful phenomenon, but it does not have to be if we properly prepare for it. For example, according to the American Council on Exercise, we begin to lose 3-10 percent of our muscles every 10 years after the age of 25.[12] This is sarcopenia. Knowing this fact, it would be wise to include resistance training as a part of a fitness program. Exercise is beneficial to the body at any age or phase: "Several recent studies have reported significant strength gains in previously sedentary older adults following a program of regular exercise, so it is never too late to begin one."[13] The aging process is one we should embrace.

4. How are you preparing to embrace the aging process?

_____

_____

5. What is sarcopenia? How can it be prevented?

_____

_____

FITNESS TIP: Aerobic training, such as walking, running, swimming, biking) will stimulate the heart and the lungs, making them more efficient. Strength training will help grow and maintain muscles. There is a saying that goes like this: "if you don't use it, you lose it." This maxim is true for muscles. If we do not use them, we will lose them and quickly too as we age.

In striving to attain optimum fitness, I have learned how important it is to marry aerobics and weight training; they are like husband and wife. Once this concept is understood, it becomes easier to see the results you want from your body.

Benefits of Weight Training

Weight training will help burn fat. Muscle tissue burns more calories than body fat, even when the body is at rest. If you are one of those individuals with a sit-down job, then you would appreciate knowing this: even while you are sitting, you are burning calories.

Weight training will build stronger bones and help ward off osteoporosis. Because bone follows function, it is important to practice good form when exercising. Solicit the help of a personal training if you can to make sure exercises are carried out correctly.

Weight training will help prevent injuries. Just as a house needs repairs and maintenance, your body will as well. Weight training helps to keep the structure strong and sturdy. As people age, many complain about falls. Weight training is one way to prevent them from occurring.

Weight training will improve body image. Tighten up those muscles. A toned body unquestionably looks better than a flabby one. More women would see results in this area when they remove the fear of getting too bulky.

Weight training leads to a higher rate in metabolism because muscles burn more calories than fat. Resistance training reverses the natural decline in metabolism after age 30. If you are one of those women over 30 and running your heart out to keep off menopausal weight, you may want to incorporate weight training. Or, if you are one of those men encountering a midlife crisis, now is the time to "beef it up"!

Weight training has a positive effect on insulin resistance. Removing carbohydrates completely out of a diet in order to lose weight is a common mistake a lot of people make. The body needs carbohydrates. Carbohydrates are the body's preferred fuel, but too much of this fuel is stored into excess fat when not used. In weight training, however, muscles need the energy from glucose (sugar) which carbohydrates are converted into. When the body converts carbohydrates into this sugar called glucose, it is stored in the muscles as glycogen. When you are training your muscles, it is this uptake of glycogen that is used.

Weight training also has a positive effect on cholesterol levels. It helps to increase the good cholesterol (high density lipoprotein) and decrease the bad cholesterol (low density lipoprotein).

41

6. Choose one of the benefits of weight training. Which one would you like to gain and why?

_____

_____

Aging Gracefully

Before we leave this chapter on our parental roots and aging, this would make a good segue to talk also about antioxidants which are believed to be vitamins that slow down the aging process. These vitamins, minerals, and other nutrients protect and repair cells from damage caused by free radicals. It is purported that these free radicals are what cause us to age and to develop chronic diseases such as cancer by attacking the cells of our bodies. The body responds by sending antioxidants to terminate the free radicals. These macronutrients cannot be manufactured by the body; they must be attained in the diet:[14]

> **Vitamin E**: d-alpha tocopherol. A fat-soluble vitamin present in nuts, seeds, vegetable and fish oils, whole grains (esp. wheat germ), fortified cereals, and apricots. Current recommended daily allowance (RDA) is 15 IU per day for men and 12 IU per day for women.

> **Vitamin C**: Ascorbic acid is a water-soluble vitamin present in citrus fruits and juices, green peppers, cabbage, spinach, broccoli, kale, cantaloupe, kiwi, and strawberries. The RDA is 60 mg per day. Intake above 2000 mg may be associated with adverse side effects in some individuals.

> **Beta-carotene** is a precursor to vitamin A (retinol) and is present in liver, egg yolk, milk, butter, spinach, carrots, squash, broccoli, yams, tomato, cantaloupe, peaches, and grains. Because beta-carotene is converted to vitamin A by the body, there is no set requirement. Instead the RDA is expressed as retinol equivalents (RE) to clarify the relationship. (NOTE: Vitamin A has no antioxidant properties and can be quite toxic when taken in excess.)

7. Circle the best answer.

Which food is recommended as a source for vitamin E?
   a. tomato

   b. cabbage

   c. fish oil

   d. green peppers

Which food is recommended as a source for beta-carotene?
   a. yams

   b. peaches

   c. cantaloupe

   d. all of the above

What is ascorbic acid?
   a. vitamin C

   b. vitamin E

   c. vitamin A

   d. none of the above

Which food can I attain both Vitamin C and Beta-carotene?
   a. seeds

   b. kiwi

   c. apricot

   d. broccoli

I truly believe that when we eat foods of life we gain life—longevity. We certainly may not live as long as Methuselah, but we, too, can benefit from eating more of the foods our loving Father created for us, His Children.

8. How does the fifth commandment protect your health and well-being?

_____

_____

Application:

Strength for your Journey and Staying Hydrated

Training like an Athlete

Weight training can boost your strength, tone your muscles, and help you lose fat. If you already workout with weights, keep it up! If you do not, add some hand weights as you walk. If you are uncomfortable about using weights, hire a personal trainer to help you get started.

Ready to start a weight-training program?

If you do not have access to a gym and its facility, then it will help to be creative. For weights you can use cans or water or milk bottles filled with water or sand.

In working out, work your big muscles first. They are the muscles in the legs, back, chest, and shoulders. The smaller muscles, such as your biceps, triceps, and calves, should be worked afterwards.

Goal:	Strength building
Number of Exercises	4 exercises that challenge all major muscle groups
Sets	3-4 sets for each exercise
Repetition	8-12 repetitions per exercise
Rest/recovery	1-2 minutes between sets
Frequency	2-3 times per week for excellent gains in strength

Choose a weight or resistance level heavy enough to tire your muscles after about 12 repetitions. Also remember your RPE (See *Ten Guiding Lights to Health and Wholeness* book). How hard are you working out?

Hydrating the Body

The human body is made up of 60% water. That's more than half. **Muscles are made up of 75% water.** Bones and fat are composed of 50% water. Drinking adequate amount of water is extremely important in order to carry out the necessary functions of the body.

Divide your weight in half. That is the number of ounces you must consume in a day. For example, if you weigh 200 pounds, you would drink 100 ounces of water. Upon arising, drink at least 32 oz. water with lemon or lime. Continue drinking throughout the day to reach your goal. That means taking your bottle with you wherever you go.

Don't forget to record your daily intake of water. (See appendix B)

Reasons for drinking water:

1. Removes wastes
2. Regulates body temperature
3. Carries nutrients and oxygen to the cells
4. Cushions and lubricates your joints and muscles
5. Dissolves nutrients to make them available to the body
6. Aids in weight loss

Ideas:

- Add lemon to your water (Lemon is a powerful antioxidant, which helps to detoxify the body.)
- Make a smoothie rich in antioxidants (Use kale, spinach, carrots, and fruits to sweeten.)

Shopping List:
- 32 oz. or more BPA-free bottle/stainless steel bottle
- Brita kitchen pitcher/faucet filtration

☑ **Checking In:**

Submit your food journal to your accountability partner. See appendix B.

Keep a record of your daily exercise. See appendix C. Remember to walk as much as possible even if you are fit and healthy.

Reflection (in your journal):
How did your relationship with your parent(s) affect your well-being? Or paint a picture in words how you would like to age.

Notes:

1. Robert Kirschner, *Divine Things: Seeking the Sacred in a Secular Age* (New York: The Crossroad Publishing Company, 2001), 124.
2. Kirschner, *Divine Things*, 124.
3. Curt Thompson, *Anatomy of the Soul: Surprising Connections between Neuroscience and Spiritual Practices That Can Transform Your Life and Relationships* (Carol Stream, IL: Tyndale House Publishers, 2010), 110, Kindle edition.
4. Thompson, *Anatomy of the Soul*, 110.
5. Ephesians 3:17.
6. David Benner, *The Gift of Being Yourself: The Sacred Call to Self-Discovery*, 80, Kindle edition.
7. Romans 8:38-39 (NIV).
8. 1 Corinthians 13:11.
9. Thompson, *Anatomy of the Soul*, 116, Kindle edition.
10. Kara Davis, *Spiritual Secrets to Weight Loss* (Lake Mary, FL: Siloam, 2008), 60.
11. Kirschner, *Divine Things: Seeking the Sacred in a Secular Age*, 122.
12. *ACE Personal Trainer Manual* (San Diego, CA: American Council on Exercise, 2003), 361.
13. *ACE Personal Trainer Manual*, 361.
14. "Antioxidants and Free Radicals." Accessed: June 2010, www.rice.edu/~jenky/sports/antiox.html.

Chapter 6

Do Not Obstruct the Flow of Life

"You must not murder."

Goals:
Understand the impact of anger
Aim to exercise for at least 150 minutes each week
Develop a holistic attitude toward health and wellness
Improve our interpersonal and intrapersonal communication
Understand how the sixth commandment protects and restores our health and well being

Objectives:
Choose life-generating words
Understand that both my thought-language and spoken words govern my behavior
Create and repeat affirmations based on scripture to alter one's thought-language
Choose one of the following goals above to focus on for the week

Your goal for this week:

_____

_____

There were two brothers named Cain and Abel. They were the children of Adam and Eve. Cain was responsible for cultivating the land, and Abel was responsible for taking care of the flock. Cain offered the fruit of the ground and Abel offered from his flock a sheep or goat as a sacrifice to God. However, God was more pleased with Abel's gift than with Cain's.

Read Genesis 4:1-16.

1. Why was God pleased with Abel's gift and displeased with Cain's?

_____

_____

2. Because God had favor on Abel, how did Cain feel?

_____

_____

3. How did this emotion affect Cain?

_____

_____

4. Jesus later expounded on the sixth commandment by including anger that is expressed in the heart and through spoken words. Read Matthew 5:21-22.

   How can anger be expressed in the heart?

_____

_____

5. According to Jesus in Matthew 5:21, why is it dangerous to harbor anger in the heart?

_____

_____

6. In *The Ten Guiding Lights*, it is said that anger can affect us physically, emotionally and socially. Give an example of each situation.

   a. Physically:

_____

_____

   b. Emotionally:

_____

_____

c. Socially:

_____

_____

_____

7. It is not wrong to be angry. But how we deal with our anger is the determining factor. According to Ephesians 4:26-27, how should we deal with our anger?

_____

_____

_____

_____

In Matthew 21:12, we see Jesus angrily overturning the tables of vendors who were selling in the temple, and driving them out. We can use anger as a motivating force to bring about positive change, as Jesus demonstrated. Or we can use anger negatively to bring about evil, such as the murder in the case of Cain. We are to be on guard or on the alert when it comes to anger, because anger can master us if we allow it (Genesis 4:7).

Words We Speak Out Loud

There is another type of murder that is both emotional and spiritual.

8. Write out Proverbs 18:21.

_____

_____

When we slander someone, badmouth a sister or brother, or say unkind words, we are actually expressing a form of murder. Some call this act character assassination. The spirit of an individual can be crushed. Proverbs 17:22 says, "a crushed spirit dries up the bones." Red blood cells are manufactured in the marrow which is found in the bones.

9. What happens if our bones dry up? What is bone marrow? What is its purpose? How does this metaphor pertaining to the body help us to understand Proverbs 17:22?

_____

_____

_____

_____

Words We Speak to Ourselves

Words are powerful. For that reason, we should think before we speak because the right words can crush a spirit. Likewise, the words we speak to ourselves can also be detrimental to our body, mind and spirit. Changing our language-based thoughts in our brains from one of fear to love requires practice and attention if we are going to experience the abundant life promised to us. What are your thoughts about your body? What are your thoughts about eating healthy? What are your thoughts about exercising? What are your thoughts about growing old? What are your thoughts about you? If you continually tell yourself you do not like exercise or you can't find the time to exercise, then these thoughts are working on your behalf. If you continually tell yourself you do not like the way you look, then these thoughts are working on your behalf. If you continually tell yourself you cannot afford healthy food, then these thoughts are working on your behalf. If you continually tell yourself you are a loser, then these thoughts are working on your behalf. The body hears, and the body listens. The body seeks to carry out what it hears from you. The answers to these questions are currently running your life.

Read Proverbs 4:23 from the New Century Version:

"Be careful what you think, because your thoughts run your life."

Certain thoughts can be very resistant to change. However, as believers we have to uproot old ways of thinking about our life in order to make space for a new way of thinking. We have to learn how to apply the Word of God to everyday living. Developing **positive affirmations** can help strengthen our identity and purpose in life, bringing a new way of thinking along with life-satisfaction and joy.

10. What are your thoughts about exercising? Do you make time for it? Why or why not?

_____

_____

_____

_____

_____

11. What are your thoughts about eating healthily? Do you do it sometimes, all the time or never?

_____

_____

_____

_____

_____

12. God has given us an authority card that defines our identity, meaning and value. Supply a scripture next to each descriptor. Then, write out the scripture reference below. The first one has been done for you.

Identity	Meaning	Value	Scripture
God's beloved	A child of God; created in God's image	Priceless	**Genesis 1:27**
Co-ruler	Restores God's rulership; takes care of the planet	Placed above all God's creation	
Heir	Recipient to all that God is	Royalty	
Co-partner	Works alongside with Christ	Calls you His Friend	
Co-creator	Ability to create & produce	Purposeful; potent	

13. Now write out your scriptures here.

God's beloved:

_____

_____

Co-ruler:

_____

_____

Heir:

_____

_____

Co-partner:

_____

_____

Co-creator:

_____

_____

Repeat the following Ten Guiding Lights affirmations *daily*:

- I am God's beloved child, co-ruler on this Earth to restore God's rulership and to care for His planet.
- I am heir of God's Kingdom. I seek his Kingdom out of which all other things are given to me.
- I am a co-laborer with Christ, responsible for sharing the gospel of health to all.
- I am a co-partner of Christ's. I have all that I need to live a healthy and a satisfying life. This is my divine health insurance.
- I am a co-creator. I think, speak and act according to what the Holy Spirit shows and tells me. I have the ability to recreate my world through my thought-based language and the words I speak.

When we speak affirmations, we speak in the present not in the future or past. We believe we are healthy not will be healthy or were healthy. This is faith, calling "things that are not as though they were (Romans 4:17, KJV). We grow our faith when we can hear God's words of life (Romans 10:17). However, we must support our faith with works, knowing it is God who will bless our efforts. Our faith should be accompanied by action according to James 2:17. If we believe we are healthy, what are we doing to support our faith?

Eating healthily and exercising consistently are two ways.

14. Write FIVE affirmations about eating healthily and end each sentence with "faith without works is dead." The first one has been done for you:

    a. I choose to eat vegetables with each meal because I want a healthy body, and faith without works is dead.

    b.

    c.

    d.

    e.

15. Write FIVE affirmations about exercising and end each sentence with "faith without works is dead." The first one has been done for you:

    a. I go to the gym rain or shine because I want a healthy body, and faith without works is dead.

    b.

    c.

    d.

    e.

Changing your thought-language for the Journey

Repeat daily your <u>personal</u> health and wellness affirmations. To bring about further change, add the *Ten Guiding Lights* affirmations.

Checking In:

Submit your food journal to your accountability partner. See appendix B.

Keep a record of your daily exercise. See appendix C. Remember to walk as much as possible even if you are fit and healthy.

Reflection (in your journal):
What are some of your predominant thoughts you repeatedly speak to yourself? Are these thoughts affecting your health and well-being?

Chapter 7

Don't Cheat Yourself by Cheating on God

"You must not commit adultery."

Goals:

Understand the role pleasure plays in our lives

Understand how food can be considered adulterous

Understand the significance of gut health

Aim to exercise for at least 150 minutes each week

Develop a holistic attitude toward health and wellness

Understand how the seventh commandment protects and restores our health and well being

Objectives:

Redefine sacrifice

Exercise at an appropriate level

Commit to a fitness and nutrition goal

Include foods that promote gut health

Demonstrate sacrificial living in making healthier choices

Your Fitness goal for this week:

_____

_____

Your Nutrition goal for this week:

_____

_____

To many believers, food has become safe sex. Proverbs says, "Food eaten in secret tastes the best!"[1] Whether eaten in secret or not, the statistics pertaining to church obesity is revealing, alarming and of grave concern. Are we finding that much pleasure in eating? Or are we eating to assuage our pain? Are we enjoying a sedentary life to the detriment of our health and well-being? Have we been deceived? Are we as the Body of Christ in an adulterous relationship with food?

1. What is the relationship between Christ and His church? Read Ephesians 5:22-23.

_____

_____

2. The book of Song of Solomon expresses a love relationship between a man and woman. In chapter 1, what does this love relationship symbolize?

_____

_____

God has strong feelings towards us. Yes, I did say feelings. He is deeply impacted by us not in a way that would affect Him as God, but in the way He responds to us. We were created for His pleasure and with the ability to enjoy pleasure. Though God has created us with this ability, we must not be deceived by it. Too much pleasure numbs us spiritually, which explains why many of us, including believers are walking around like dead people.

3. Timothy, an apostle of Jesus Christ, describes a widow who indulged in pleasure as _____ although she was _____ (1Timothy 5:6).

God wants us to experience pleasure. But pleasure attained without discipline is an illusion. Food can be such an illusion. In the absence of restraint, we can attain great pleasure from food instantaneously. Food, for some, can be as or more pleasurable than sex.

Specifically, carbohydrates, such as chips, cakes, cookies, ice cream, candies, pasta, breads, alcohol, and rice can tend to be pleasurable and thus addictive, because they are comforting. They have the power to soothe, calm, and relax us. As a result, we call such carbohydrates **comfort foods**. They are also mainly processed foods (foods that have been altered from their natural state). When some people are stressed, bored, or depressed, they consume these foods in excess amounts. As we have learned, carbohydrates affect the levels of our blood sugar. These particular foods quickly release so much sugar into the blood that the body counteracts the increase by releasing the hormone insulin which triggers the fat cells.

Neurologically, this connection between emotions and food occurs in the brain. The brain contains neurotransmitters—hormones made from amino acids, which are responsible for controlling movements, certain emotional response, and the physical ability to feel pleasure and pain. We experience a rise in endorphins, "feel good" hormones, during and after exercise. When we are low in endorphins, we might cry for no apparent reason and become overly sensitive. Another neurotransmitter is serotonin. If our serotonin level is low, then we tend to become negative, obsessive, worried, irritable, and sleepless. On the other hand, if we are high in serotonin, we tend to be optimistic, confident, flexible, and easygoing. Catecholamine, another neurotransmitter, can also affect us emotionally. If this hormone level is low, then we can fall into a flat, lethargic funk. Then, if we are stressed and overwhelmed, low levels of the neurotransmitter GABA (gamma-aminobutyric acid) can affect us negatively. But if we have the right balance, then we are relaxed and stress-free.

Having a balanced diet consisting of proteins (amino acids), complex carbohydrates (whole grains and starches), vegetables (fibrous carbohydrates), and fruits will help us maintain a healthy emotional state so that it is easier to pray and meditate and to exercise, rest, and relax while in this body.

Though there are some factors we cannot control, we need to be vigilant that the gut does not become a portal from which strongholds come and set up camp.

How enlightening that in the Hebrew the word translated "belly"—*beten*—is used geographically and figuratively to express the various activities of neurotransmitters.

Trust Your Gut Instinct

Circle the answer that best expresses the meaning of "belly" in each scripture:

4. Surely he shall not feel quietness in his **belly**, he shall not save of that which he desired (Job 20:20 KJV).

   a. **Hungry for more food**
   b. **Emotional unrest**

5. The spirit of man is the candle of the LORD, searching all the inward parts of the **belly** (Proverbs 20:27 KJV).

   a. **The brain/mind/soul**
   b. **The large intestine/small intestine/gall bladder**

6. The words of a talebearer are as wounds, and they go down into the innermost parts of the **belly** (Proverbs 18:8 KJV).

   a. **Inner being**
   b. **Outer being**

7. He that believeth on me, as the scripture hath said, out of his **belly** shall flow rivers of living water. [But this spake he of the Spirit, which they that believe on him should receive: for the Holy Ghost was not yet given; because that Jesus was not yet glorified.] (John 7:38 KJV)

   a. **Place from which fresh water flows**
   b. **Place from which the Holy Spirit flows**

It should be of no surprise, then, that gut health determines the health of our entire being—body, mind and spirit. If our foods are not properly digested, or if our body cannot probably absorb the nutrients from foods in the small intestine, then the remainder of the body cannot receive the nutrition to function adequately. Foods with live probiotics help keep the environment of the gut healthy, so that the nutrients from foods can be absorbed. Healthy foods, particularly "living foods," contain life and thus energy. They aid and support our whole being in carrying out certain activities whether physical, mental or spiritual, so that we can flow with ease prayerfully, spiritually, creatively, intellectually, mindfully, and physically.

Some foods that keep the environment of the gut healthy are listed below:

- Foods rich in probiotics: live-probiotics, kefir, kombucha tea, kimchi, sauerkraut, pickles
- Good carbs mainly fibrous vegetables and high quality fats such as, olive oil, nuts
- Dark chocolate, coffee, wine (in moderation) and tea (to your heart's content)
- Foods rich in prebiotics: raw garlic, cooked and raw onions, leeks, jicama
- Filtered water

8. What are comfort foods? Do you eat any comfort foods? Give 3 examples of comfort foods? When do you normally eat these foods?

_____

_____

_____

_____

9. Name 4 neurotransmitters. Explain their function.

a. _____

b. _____

c _____

d. _____

Food, Exercise and the Spiritual Journey
Food, therefore, can aid us on our spiritual journey or it can be an impasse. How do we know it can be an impasse?

10. Read Matthew 6:17-18. What did Jesus encourage his disciples to do?

_____

_____

The act of fasting helps in disciplining the body. Unless we discipline our bodies, in other words, delay pleasure periodically, we will not achieve God's promise of a healthy life.

The act of exercising is another way of disciplining the body. Getting up early in the morning to exercise can be considered a sacrifice for many. For others, it could be working out in the evening after a long exhausting day at work. Or adhering to a healthy diet throughout the week can also be considered a sacrifice, especially after a stressful day when the body yearns for foods high in carbohydrates instead. These choices can all be considered sacrifices because they result in some type of discomfort by delaying pleasure. Perhaps, then, for some, the mere act of exercising is a sacrifice, especially when the body is already in pain. When we make sacrifices unto God as Daniel did, God sees our acts and honors them.

Here is some additional information to help you judge your exercise intensity from the Mayo Foundation for Medical Education and Research (2011):[2]

Light exercise intensity

Light activity feels easy. Here are clues that your exercise intensity is at a light level:
- You have no noticeable changes in your breathing pattern.
- You don't break a sweat (unless it's very hot or humid).
- You can easily carry on a full conversation or even sing.

Ideal for taking leisurely walks, especially with your dog.

Moderate exercise intensity (somewhat hard)

Moderate activity feels somewhat hard. Here are clues that your exercise intensity is at a moderate level:
- Your breathing quickens, but you're not out of breath.
- You develop a light sweat after about 10 minutes of activity.
- You can carry on a conversation, but you can't sing.

Ideal for working out.

Vigorous exercise intensity (hard)

Vigorous activity feels challenging. Here are clues that your exercise intensity is at a vigorous level:
- Your breathing is deep and rapid.
- You develop a sweat after a few minutes of activity.
- You can't say more than a few words without pausing for breath.

Sometimes the body needs a change but not encouraged for a long period of time. Special care must be taken to avoid injury.

Overexerting yourself (extremely hard)
Beware of pushing yourself too hard too often. If you are short of breath, in pain, or can't work out as long as you had planned, your exercise intensity is probably higher than your fitness level allows. Back off a bit, and build intensity gradually.

Like most disciplines, exercise initially is not pleasurable. The pleasure comes as we continue to practice or exercise. God has given us wonderful hormones called endorphins to motivate us.

Application:
Exercise

- Sign up for at least a 5k walk/ race.
- Practice every day for it.
- Make sure you are in the moderate to vigorous zone.

Nutrition: Kill two birds with one stone

Eat carbohydrates that would promote **gut health, supply fiber, and help in weight loss or maintenance.**

These foods will do all of the above:
Sweet potato
Brown rice
Quinoa
Oatmeal
Barley
Lentil
Add some garlic and leeks to your pot.

"Basically, all that grows in God's garden is perfect for the body."

Resistant Starch and Gut Health

Resistant starch is a type of dietary fiber naturally found in potatoes, grains and beans, particularly when these foods are cooled. Cooling either at room temperature or in the refrigerator will turn these carbohydrates into resistant starch. When these starches become resistant, they act like fiber, going through the stomach and small intestine undigested. For this reason, they do not cause a rise in blood sugar levels. They also feed the friendly bacteria in the large intestine needed to keep the gut healthy.

Here are some ideas to try:

- Substitute hummus for mayo
- Cold or room temperature
  - Potato, Barley, Lentil, Brown rice salad
  - Green banana (delicious when boiled)
  - Brown rice pudding
- Raw oats (try a bowl of muesli)

Always practice portion control with everything.

Checking In:

Submit your food journal to your accountability partner. See appendix B.

Keep a record of your daily exercise. See appendix C. Remember to walk as much as possible even if you are fit and healthy.

Reflection (in your journal):
Where are some places you find solace? Are these places healthy for your well-being? Why or why not?

Notes:

1. Proverbs 9:17.
2. Mayo Foundation for Medical Education and Research, *Exercise intensity: Why it matters, how it's measured,* Accessed May, 2011. Retrieved from www.mayoclinic.com/ health/exercise-intensity/SM00113/.

Chapter 8

Don't Steal God's Glory

"You must not steal."

Goals:
Develop a holistic attitude toward health and wellness
Aim to exercise for at least 150 minutes each week
Honor my body as a sacred living temple for God's glory
Make a commitment to a fitness, nutrition, and wellness goal
Understand the importance of carrying God's glory within my body
Understand how the eighth commandment protects and restores our health and well being

Objectives:
Distinguish between false and true self
Apply concept of the false and true self myself
Offer forgiveness to myself or someone else
Commit to a fitness, nutrition, and wellness goal

Your Fitness goal for this week:

_____

_____

Your Nutrition goal for this week:

_____

_____

Your Wellness goal for this week:

_____

_____

A dam and Eve believed the serpent. Eve "saw that the tree was good for food, that it was pleasant to the eyes, and a tree desirable to make one wise," so she ate the fruit and gave it also to her husband. Their eyes were both opened, and "they knew that they were naked," so "they sewed fig leaves together and made themselves coverings."[1] Adam and Eve wanted to be like God without God. Because Adam and Eve attempted to steal from God His glory, their bodies were covered with shame. The fig leaves became a symbolic representation of their shame.

When we attempt to 'do life' without God, all we receive is an illusion.

The body is God's glory. It has been redeemed. However, our former or false nature can still live out of this body at the expense of the true self or the "new man." The true self lives out of its new life."[2] It is the true self that is defined by Christ. And it is the true self that brings health and healing to the body. This is transformation from the inside-out.

1. In Romans 6:6, what does the Apostle Paul call the false nature?

_____

_____

The false nature, which will be addressed as the false self from here on, can affect our sense of well-being. The false self has to upkeep and protect an image, and this in itself creates stress for the body. It is the false self that seeks to rob God of His glory, whereas the true self seeks to bring glory to God. The following statements represent the "true self".

The body is God's Creation. The body is a part of God's wonderful creation. Like nature which declares God's glory, (Psalm 19:1) the body is made to display God's beauty as well (1 Corinthians 6:20a). Just as nature points to God, our actions, words and thoughts should point to God too (Ephesians 2:10; Matthew 5:16).

Be vulnerable. Vulnerability is uncomfortable. We expose the good and bad to God. As the song says, it's coming to God "just as I am."[3] Since God already knows us, why try to perform?

Love your body. God does not "dwell in temples made with human hands" (Acts 7:48a). He also lives within our body—His Kingdom is within us (Luke 17:21). We love our body because it is a sacred space that was purchased with His life.

Be grounded in God's love. Apostle Paul encouraged us to be rooted in Christ's love. God is love. We know God through His love. Through His love, He transforms us.

Be real and 'be' in love. Because we are loved by God, we do not have to pretend to be strong. We can find our strength in Christ instead. It is in Christ we are strong.

Be humble. In God's kingdom, promotion is from the ground up. New life can grow out of our brokenness. Our pain can bring about humility and, as a result, allow space for God (John 3:30).

Receive your identity, value, meaning and dignity from God. God has given us dominion to operate with Him as co-creator, co-partner, co-laborer, and co-regent on the earth. He establishes our identity; His name is written on our foreheads (Revelation 22:4). He gives us value; we are bought with His blood—priceless (1 Corinthians 6:20). He gives us meaning; we are born to do good works for the honor and glory of His name (Ephesians 2:10). We are created in God's image; no one can take away our dignity.

Embrace your weakness and strength. As human beings, we are imperfect; there is good and bad in us. Apostle Paul recognized that there were two opposing sides within him: the one that wanted to do good but did not and the other that did what was wrong (Romans 7:15). We have to accept ourselves as is and surrender ourselves to God's love. We cannot give to God what we have not fully accepted.

2. Read the statements below. If a statement represents you truthfully, write the letter "T" on the line next to it. If a statement represents you falsely, write the letter "F" on the line next to it.

_____ I accept my strengths as well as my weaknesses.

_____ I hide my weaknesses and embrace only my strengths.

_____ I am my own creation; "I seek glory for myself."

_____ I exist to bring God glory.

_____ I must present my best self, whatever that may mean, on the stage of life.

_____ I surrender to God my weaknesses and strengths.

_____ I own my space—my body.

_____ My body belongs to God. Within me, the Holy Spirit lives.

——— I will allow myself to be filled with God's love, and this love will bring about my transformation.

_____ I am rooted in myself. "I bring about my own transformation."

_____ I can be open and honest before God who knows and sees the real person I am.

_____ I pretend to be strong and I wear a mask.

_____ C. S. Lewis expressed it best: "True humility is not thinking less of yourself; it is thinking of yourself less."

_____ Exaggerates the self always; elevates the self.

_____ I create my own identity, value, and meaning and dignity or I use other people's measuring stick to determine them.

_____ It is God who gives me identity, value, meaning and dignity. No one can take these away.

When we focus on the self without God, we can become self-fixated, never discovering the true beautiful and gracious self that is defined by God.

3. In Colossians 3:12-15, how does God define the true and gracious self?

_____

_____

_____

We rob God of his glory when we do not live with a focus on Him. We become so big in our eyes that there is no room for the Holy Spirit. Understanding ourselves in the context of God puts us, His creation, into perspective. As David asked, who are we that God would be mindful of us? In relation to the universe—its galaxy with trillions of stars—Planet Earth appears as only a speck.[4] Yet God chooses to place us humans—the zenith of His creation— there. We are the apple of His eye, His beloved.

We have to know how God sees us, for it is God who knows the true self, not the self we have created.

4. Based on your responses to question 2, how do you see yourself? Begin here and continue in your journal.

_____

_____

_____

_____

_____

_____

_____

_____

_____

_____

In seeking to rob God of His glory, we all fell short of His glorious ideal, according to Romans 3:23.

5. Why did we fall short of God's standard?

_____

_____

6. Based on Isaiah 42:8, what are the two (2) things God says He will not do?

_____

_____

King Nebuchadnezzar learned this lesson the hard way.

King Nebuchadnezzar's power grew throughout the earth. His kingdom and dominion were matchless. Nebuchadnezzar was undoubtedly proud of his achievements, declaring his success as the work he did with own "mighty power" and for the honor of his great "majesty." While these words were still in Nebuchadnezzar's mouth, he lost his kingdom and his sanity. Deranged, Nebuchadnezzar was driven from society to live with beasts of the field. He ate the grass like oxen; his body was wet with the dew of heaven till his hair had grown like eagles' feathers and his nails like birds' claws.⁵ Nebuchadnezzar was humiliated and humbled by God.

After Nebuchadnezzar's time of suffering had ended, he came to his senses.

7. Read Daniel chapter 4. What was Nebuchadnezzar's conclusion after he regained his mind?

_____

_____

Pride—our own arrogance—can affect our health. Nebuchadnezzar's refusal to acknowledge the greatness of God cost him his mental state—a complete disconnect from his soul, people, reality and God. Acknowledging God's presence is important to Him for the mere fact that He is God, the One who sustains life.

Carrying God's Glory
The ancient Hebrews carried God's glory in the ark. Only priests were allowed to touch this sacred object with poles extending on each side to avoid direct contact.⁶ Later, Solomon built a temple to house God's presence.⁷ Today, God's Spirit lives within us in order that He may bring glory to the Father.

8. **Complete the blanks with the correct scriptures.**

In 1 Corinthians 10:31, everything we do including _____ or _____ should be

done for the _____ of God. Ephesians 2: 10 states we are God's _____,

created in Christ Jesus to do _____ _____, which God prepared in

advance for us to do. These acts, according to Matthew 5:16, allow our _____ to

shine so that others may _____ our Father in heaven. We exist for God's glory.

Just as the _____ declare the glory of God and the skies

_____ the work of his hands (Psalm 19:1), we are to acknowledge God

in everything we do.

9. What does it mean to you to be created for God's glory?

_____

_____

Application:

God wants to help us in everything we do? What are your health and wellness goals? In what ways will you give Him the glory? Here are some examples.

Fitness

- Will you commit to a 5k walk/run?
- Will you commit to walking during every lunch break?
- Will you commit to walking your dog at least once a day?
- Will you commit to taking the stairs or parking at a reasonable distance when it is within your power and strength to walk?

Nutrition

- Will you commit to eating a salad every day?
- Will you commit to eating only one comfort food a week?
- Will you commit to eating at least 4 servings of vegetable and 1-2 servings of fruit each day?
- Will you drink the recommended ounces of water for your body weight even when you are not thirsty?

Wellness

- Are you holding a grudge? Have you forgiven yourself or someone?
- Are you too prideful to share your weaknesses or hurts?
- Will you commit to eradicating any addictive behavior (such as smoking or pornography) or seeking out help (such as a recovery program, a spiritual director or counselor)?
- Will you commit to taking time out to answer the journal questions and to pray to God about your needs and desires if you have not done so already?

Checking In:

Submit your food journal to your accountability partner. See appendix B.

Keep a record of your daily exercise. See appendix C. Remember to walk as much as possible even if you are fit and healthy.

Reflection (in your journal):
Question number two asked you to identify each statement as true or false if you personally identified with it. Now reexamine the correct answers to each statement in the True/False Self chart below. How do you see yourself based on the chart and your responses to question number two?

True/False Self Chart

False Self **True Self**	➢ I am my own creation; "I seek glory for myself." ➢ I exist to bring God glory.
False Self **True Self**	➢ I must present my best self, whatever that may mean, on the stage of life. ➢ I surrender to God my weaknesses and strengths.
False Self **True Self**	➢ I own my space—my body. ➢ My body belongs to God. Within me, the Holy Spirit lives.
False Self **True Self**	➢ I am rooted in myself. "I bring about my own transformation." ➢ I will allow myself to be filled with God's love, and this love will bring about my transformation.
False Self **True Self**	➢ I pretend to be strong and I wear a mask. ➢ I can be open and honest before God who knows and sees the real person I am.
False Self **True Self**	➢ Exaggerates the self always; elevates the self. ➢ C. S. Lewis expressed it best: "True humility is not thinking less of yourself; it is thinking of yourself less."
False Self **True Self**	➢ I create my own identity, value, and meaning and dignity, or I use other people's measuring stick to determine them. ➢ It is God who gives me identity, value, meaning and dignity. No one can take these away.
False Self **True Self**	➢ I hide my weaknesses and embrace only my strengths. ➢ I accept my strengths as well as my weaknesses.

Notes:

1. Genesis 3:6-7.
2. Romans 6:13.
3. "Just As I Am" is a well-known hymn, written by Charlotte Elliott in 1835.
4. Psalm 8:3-4.

5. Daniel 4:30-33.
6. Exodus 37:1-9.
7. 2 Chronicles 1-14.

Chapter Nine

Don't Mistreat Yourself by Mistreating Your Neighbor

"You must not testify falsely against your neighbor."

Goals:
Love others as myself
Love myself as Christ loves me
Develop a holistic attitude toward health and wellness
Aim to exercise for at least 150 minutes each week
Make a commitment to a fitness, nutrition, and wellness goal
Understand how the ninth commandment protects and restores our health and well being

Objectives:
Define my neighbor
Exercise at an appropriate level
Commit to a fitness, nutrition, and wellness goal
Recognize the lies I tell myself and project onto others

Your Fitness goal for this week:

_____

_____

Your Nutrition goal for this week:

_____

_____

Your Wellness goal for this week:

_____

_____

One day a religious expert asked Jesus what must he do to inherit eternal life. Jesus replied by asking him what did the law of Moses say?

The man replied saying, "'You must love the Lord your God with all your heart, all your soul, all your strength, and all your mind.' And, 'Love your neighbor as yourself.'"

Jesus, then, told the man he was correct.

The man then asked Jesus who his neighbor was.

So Jesus told this story:

There was a Jewish man traveling from Jerusalem going to Jericho. The man was mugged and left half dead alongside the road.

It so happened that a priest came. He saw the man, looked and crossed to the other side of the road.

Later a temple assistant came. He, too, saw the man and did the same.

A Samaritan man, who was considered a lower class in the Jewish tradition, came. He saw the man, had compassion and helped him.

Jesus asked which of these men would be considered a neighbor to the man? The religious expert answered the one who showed compassion.

Jesus, then, responded: "Yes, now go and do the same."[1]

    1. According to Jesus, who is our neighbor?

_____

_____

    2. Jesus' definition of "neighbor" was considered revolutionary. Why?

_____

_____

The lies we tell ourselves and about others...
Unfortunately, we do tell lies about our neighbor because we often cast our own darkness upon them. We live in fear of being known because people may not love us if we reveal who we really are; prideful of our own accomplishments because we did it all by ourselves; jealous of our neighbor's success because we are disappointed with ourselves for not having or achieving;

ashamed of our hurt and pain because nobody else shares our experiences or we're not supposed to hurt. These lies we tell ourselves are projected onto our neighbor in the form of hatred, bigotry, racism, wars, slavery, colonialism, institutional injustices, murder, and the list goes on. Our communities are broken because we are broken. It takes a body of healthy individuals to form a healthy community. An African proverb teaches that a single bracelet does not jingle. We do not operate in isolation. Healthy living also requires a healthy community, which begins with personal transformation.

Dying to the False Self -The Inner Work

This journey to healthy living begins from within—the way we perceive ourselves. When we are unable to accept and love ourselves fully, we tend to be overly critical, and extremely sensitive and judgmental of others.

Like Adam and Eve, our natural tendency is to cover our flaws rather than face them. But we must face these defects in our character if we are to give them to God, for that walk of humanity from Jerusalem to Calvary gave us the model of what it was to be human—how to love God, how to love ourselves, how to love one another, and how to deal with the vicissitudes of life despite the imperfections surrounding us and our world.

3. According to Matthew 22:37, how are we to love God?

_____

_____

4. This love for God is the greatest commandment. What is the second greatest commandment as stated in Matthew 22:39?

_____

_____

Sometimes, it is hard for us to love ourselves because of what we see within us. We even speak untruths to ourselves, listening to the "father of lies" (John 8:44) rather than to the voice of God which is life. Although we are now "new creatures" (2 Corinthians 5:17), change for most of us is a process not an overnight experience. Instead of loving from a starting point from within, we love from a Christ *centeredness.*

5. Write out the new commandment given according to John 13:34?

_____

_____

_____

_____

6. Why is the new commandment more powerful than the second? Explain. According to this new commandment, to what degree do we now love ourselves and others?

_____

_____

_____

The new commandment encompasses the first. Christ models the perfected love for us. We, in return, demonstrate this perfect love Christ has shown us by loving ourselves and others. The agape love is the highest form of love we can attain and share.

Dying to Your Neighbor - Not Judging

For some, before they can focus on living a healthy life, the bleeding of their heart has to be stopped first. We are to be "Samaritans" to our neighbors and help by showing compassion. Henri Nouwen calls this process of developing compassion dying to our neighbor; it means "to stop judging them, to stop evaluating them, and thus to become free to be compassionate."[2] Our judgments so often color the way we see people. Instead of embracing them with open arms we begin to jump to conclusions that are not necessarily true.

7. How is the Golden Rule, "[d]o to others whatever you would have them do to you," reflected in Luke 6:37-38?

_____

_____

_____

Speaking the Truth in Love

We are children of love. Paul calls us "children of the light" and "children of the day."[3] We speak the truth in love. We enlighten; we inspire; we uplift. In difficult situations, the truth is not always easy to receive but necessary for growth. However, our words should always be "seasoned with salt."[4]

8. What does it mean for your words to be described as "seasoned with salt" (Colossians 4:6) and the tongue to be described as having the "power of life and death" (Proverbs 18:21)?

_____

_____

_____

_____

Jesus demonstrated both empathy and compassion during His time here on earth, particularly in healing the sick. But there is one miracle that really stands out from the others. The story surrounding the shortest verse in the Bible, "Jesus wept."[5] This story involved the death of Mary and Martha's brother, Lazarus.

Jesus arrives late. Lazarus is dead. Jesus is emotionally moved by Lazarus' death. Perhaps he is thinking of His own future death. Jesus brings Lazarus back to life, and everybody is happy once again.

We, too, are called to enter into life fully with our neighbors—to be happy with those who are happy, and weep with those who weep.[6] As people in community, we have become very independent and isolated. Yet this is not God's design. We are to celebrate life—share in each other's sufferings and enjoy the highs of each other's life.

Application:

Being a Neighbor on Your Journey

God wants to help us in everything we do. What are your health and wellness goals? In what ways will you give Him the glory? Here are some examples:

Fitness

- Will you commit to a 5k walk/run?
- Will you commit to walking during every lunch break?
- Will you commit to walking your dog at least once a day?
- Will you commit to taking the stairs or parking at a reasonable distance when it is within your power and strength to walk?

Nutrition

- Will you commit to eating a salad every day?
- Will you commit to eating only one comfort food a week?
- Will you commit to eating at least 4 servings of vegetable and 1-2 servings of fruit each day?
- Will you drink the recommended ounces of water for your body weight even when you are not thirsty?

Wellness

- Are you holding a grudge? Have you forgiven yourself or someone?
- Are you too prideful to share your weaknesses or hurts?
- Will you commit to eradicating any addictive behavior (such as smoking or pornography) or seeking out help (such as a recovery program, a spiritual director or counselor)?

▪ Will you commit to taking time out to answer the journal questions and to pray to God about your needs and desires if you have not done so already?

✓ Checking In:

Submit your food journal to your accountability partner. See appendix B.

Keep a record of your daily exercise. See appendix C. Remember to walk as much as possible even if you are fit and healthy.

Reflection (in your journal):
Our neighbor can be anyone who needs our help. Step outside of your comfort zone and find someone you do not know to help.

How can you be a good neighbor in your community? Is there anything that prevents you from being a good neighbor?

Notes:
1. Luke 10:25-37.
2. Henri J. M. Nouwen, The Way of the Heart: Desert Spirituality and Contemporary Ministry (New York, N.Y.: The Seabury Press, 1981), 35.
3. I Thessalonians 5:5 (NIV).
4. Colossians 4:6 (NIV).
5. John 11:35.
6. Romans 12:15.

Chapter Ten

Don't Compare Yourself with Others

"You must not covet."

Goals:

Beware of a covetous mindset

Desire to be what God wants me to be

Understand what it means to covet someone else's body

Understand the importance of accepting myself wholly

Understand the integration of body, mind and spirit

Understand how activities such as exercise and meditation can integrate my being

Understand how the tenth commandment protects and restores my health and well being

Objectives:

Define covetousness

Express gratitude for my body

Recognize covetousness in everyday life

Write a personal mission statement

Commit to a fitness, nutrition, and wellness goal

Meditate on the Word of God to foster wellness and success

Your Fitness goal for this week:

_____

_____

Your Nutrition goal for this week:

_____

_____

Your Wellness goal for this week:

_____

_____

Open the door to a spirit of covetousness and we will experience a slow death that gradually seeps like a lethal poison into our being. The *Easton Bible Dictionary* defines covetousness as "a strong desire after the possession of worldly things,"[1] particularly in regards to other people's achievement or possession. The word and its definition seem antiquated, but if we understand what happens to us when we become excessively desirous of things that are transitory or when we respond with envy or resentment to our neighbor's success, then we would also comprehend why this commandment is one of the most relevant for the purpose of achieving and maintaining health and wholeness.

Covetousness is a joy killer because it sows the seed of ingratitude. Ingratitude is a negative emotion, which then breeds other dark emotions, such as envy, resentment and hatred. The opposite response to covetousness is gratitude. As people of faith, we are to be thankful for all things.[2]

1. What is covetousness?

_____

_____

2. Why is gratitude the opposite response to covetousness?

_____

_____

3. According to Exodus 20:17, what does the Bible say we should not covet?

_____

_____

_____

4. How can we apply this commandment to everyday living and to our health and wellness goals?

_____

_____

Too often we are dissatisfied with our bodies and desirous of someone else's or tempted to feel inadequate if we cannot achieve the so-called perfect body. Images in magazines, social media, online, in particular, have a powerful impact on our psyches—teens being the most vulnerable.

For these reasons, when we as believers begin to focus on the body, it is important that we do so from a place of health and with an understanding of the body's greater purpose, which is to carry out the assigned will of God. Being thankful to our Creator should then be our first response to Him for gifting us with a body. Furthermore, since God accepts us just as we are and not as we should be, we should also do likewise—accept ourselves wholly.

5. How can being aware of the spirit of covetousness protect our health and well-being as we care for the body?

_____

_____

_____

6. Name 3 things about your body for which you are thankful?

_____

_____

_____

7. Based on 3 John 1:2, what is God's desire concerning our physical health?

_____

_____

8. According to Psalm 43:5, why should believers also have a healthy disposition?

_____

_____

9. Why can social media become a breeding ground for covetousness?

_____

_____

_____

_____

10. Why do we have to be careful that our desires originate from a pure heart?

_____

_____

_____

_____

Wired for Integration—Body, Mind and Spirit

Jesus grew strong in mind and body; He grew in favor with God and men.[3] In order to become one with the mind of Christ, we have to transform our thinking.[4] This change is not limited to our spiritual life but all of life. God is concerned about what we put in our body, and what we do with our body because it belongs to Him. It is where His spirit—the Holy Spirit—is dwelling. Food, for example, is like the act of sex; it becomes one with our body. For instance, eventually, all of the processed meats we have consistently eaten can give birth in the form of cancer.[5]

Our bodies are designed to connect physically, mentally and spiritually. Physically, it unites sexually. Mentally, it unites synergistically. Spiritually, the body unites on all levels. That's why Paul speaks strongly to the church at Corinth concerning sexual sins.[6] The fact that the body is the means in which our mind and spirit connect us to life is also the reason food was such a big deal for the Hebrews. It is also the reason "naming" becomes so important to God. It is the reason the attachment to our parents can affect our relationship with God. It is the reason the words we speak have power to bring life or death. It is the reason why loving our neighbor is as important as loving oneself. It is the reason every part of our body has been redeemed. The body is the connector. It has to be addressed contextually. It has to be addressed according to God's plan for it. It has to be addressed as a sacred place belonging to the Holy Spirit. Taking care of a house requires proper management.

11. Can you give an example how our body and spirit can be united?

_____

_____

_____

Since the house—our body—does not belong to us we have to be careful with what desires, wants and wishes occupy it. That's why paying attention to our thought-life is so critical. Too many times we are distracted by external factors that may not even be the devil at work but simply our lack of ability to stay focused.

Mindfulness, which is paying attention in a particular way to the present moment, can help us be more attentive to our thought-life. Meditation is a vehicle for mindfulness, which reduces stress, improves immune functions and increases creativity, clarity, focus and efficiency at work. But most importantly, meditation is a means of training the mind. If God instructs us to meditate on His Word,[7] He is teaching us how to pay attention to it in a particular way and how to use His Word to transform our minds in order to achieve His Kingdom agenda.

Meditation is simple but not necessarily easy until we make it a practice, like prayer and reading the Word of God. When we meditate, we should:

- Observe our breath because it is the breath of God—His Holy *Ruach* (The Hebrew word for breath, wind, spirit)[8] within us.

- Observe our emotions and thoughts. We need to allow God to see our thoughts and surrender them to Him. In our weakness, His strength is perfected.

- Incorporate a scripture or a story from the Bible.

12. The Hebrew word "Ruach" means breath. When God breathed His breath into us, we became a _____ _____ (Genesis 2:7 KJV).

13. Read Joshua 1:8. How does meditation help us in training the mind?

_____

_____

_____

Connecting body and mind is natural. When we exercise, the body feels better; and, as a result, the mind function improves. When we include God in this space also, we experience more of life running through our bodies. We feel a deeper purpose for living, for we are living for a higher calling that transcends our personal life and life on this earth. We become more sensitive and aware of God's Presence in the here and now. **We are more attentive, so that there are certainly no coincidences or serendipities, but God's divine workings—miracles every day.** As believers, when we treat our body, mind and spirit as a unified entity, we are more fully equipped to deal with life, especially those difficult emotions.

Guided Meditation

1. Put your feet flat on the floor and close your eyes.
2. Sit up straight—nice and tall.
3. Notice your breath—God's breath. It is his Holy *Ruach* within you. Become aware of His presence.
4. If your mind wanders—see your thoughts and allow them to sail by like a sailboat.
5. With each exhale, release the tensions, the stress, the worries and the desires. Many times our desires create stress and tensions within us. Release them. Surrender them.

6. See yourself releasing them to God like a balloon releasing air slowing. Trust Him. Entrust them to Him. With each exhale release—let go.
7. Relax the body as you continue to breathe. Begin with your head; move down to your shoulders, your arms, legs and feet.
8. Allow this time of stillness to remind you that you are in the Presence of God. Be still and know that you are in the presence of The Most High God.
9. Bask in God's Presence. Stay here. Feel the warmth of His Presence. You are safe here in His arms.

Stay as long as you are able. You can start with 5 minutes if you have difficulty sitting still.

Wired for Integration—Embracing our Brokenness

We began with the story of Adam and Eve, so we will end with them—the beginning, where everything fell apart. Their desire to become godlike without God brought the shame and pain that's in our world today. Our brokenness is a part of who we are.[9] Many times we want to focus on simply our strengths, but in doing so we become dependent on ourselves, falling prey to the idol of perfectionism. "God wants us to be aware of our helplessness," explains Benner, "so that we can know that we need Divine help."[10]

14. In 2 Corinthians 12:9-10, the Apostle Paul is very aware of his shortcoming. Why does Paul view this weakness as a positive?

_____

_____

_____

15. How are we both God's masterpiece and a work in progress?

_____

_____

_____

Many of us are familiar with the analogy of the body to a temple, but Paul also describes us as God's masterpiece,[11] which He has created anew in Christ Jesus so we can do the good things He planned for us long ago. I like this description because it gives insight into who God is and what God thinks of us. The word masterpiece means outstanding work of art or craft; it is the greatest work of an artist. We are God's finest artistry. He is the Artist to whom we give all credit. To God, we are His beloved; we are His masterpiece and no one can undo that truth.

Loving Our Body

Therefore, learning to love our body wholly is part of the healing of our brokenness. Christ accepts us wholly, so we, too, should accept ourselves. We all have to be taught to love our bodies healthily. Yet we know more than ever that it is challenging to love our bodies in a world of Slim Fast and Jenny Craig diets, pencil-thin celebrities, plastic surgeries, and liposuctions. We have exercise gadgets, app personal trainers, group fitness classes all to motivate us to get fit. Then there are ideas about nutrition. Vegan. Paleo. Clean eating. Raw food. Take your pick. We can make all of these changes, but if we don't learn to love the body first, the changes will become temporary and non-transformational.

> **The Mirror Exercise**
> Set aside time to perform this exercise. After showering, look in the mirror at your body. This may be difficult for some, but ask the Holy Spirit to help you. Express your appreciation to God for gifting you with a body, for it allows you to remain here on Earth. Ask for forgiveness if you have not taken care of His body. Ask for His forgiveness if you have not accepted it as a gift.

Once you have accepted your body as is, SURRENDER it to Him. Be kind and compassionate to yourself as God works on you to perfect what He promised.

Our Body for His

Through Christ's sacrifice all things have been reconciled to Him. "God has brought all things back to Himself again—things on earth and things in heaven. God made peace through the blood of Christ's death on the cross."[12] Now we are able to make peace with our body by accepting the Father's love offering in Jesus. If we accept the Father's gift, then we accept the newness of life that He gives us.

The communion has come to symbolize this newness of life and unity.

Jesus takes His place at the table with His friends. Bread and wine are provided. He gives thanks for each one. He takes the bread and breaks it into pieces, saying, "This is my body, which is given for you. Do this in memory of me." Then, He shares the cup of wine with His friends, telling them, "This cup is God's new covenant sealed with my blood, which is poured out for you."[13]

We are asked by Jesus to remember this time together—to pay attention to it in a particular way, for the communion reminds us that the body is significant to God. So potent is this act upon our body that special care has to be taken to prepare for it, lest we bring sickness or death upon ourselves.[14] We are asked to examine ourselves.[15]

Guided Meditation

1. Close your eyes.
2. Become aware of your breath. Breathe deeply.
3. Like a balloon slowly releasing air, release any thought to Him.
4. Inhale and exhale about ten times again.
5. With each exhale, let go of your hurts, your worries, your cares, your fears. Slowly release your grip; relax your fingers; slowly let go. Breathe. It is His *Ruach* within you. [Pause-Breathe]
6. Now imagine you are sitting at the table with Jesus and His friends. You're in His presence.
7. See Jesus holding the bread. He breaks it into pieces, saying "This is My body, which is given for you. Do this in memory of me."
8. The bread is passed to you.
9. Slowly chew the bread. Realize that this bread is Jesus' body. His body became broken for you.
10. Jesus passes the wine to each of you. Hear him saying, "This cup is God's new covenant sealed with My blood, which is poured out for you."
11. Receive the cup from Jesus. Drink from the cup. Drink life. Drink health. Drink healing.
12. Now pass it to the next disciple.
13. See Him on the cross, His body tortured and bleeding.
14. Now see Him before you smiling.
15. Open your eyes, for He is alive.

If in a group, you can also take the actual communion if there is a leader to officiate it.

Here are some tips for staying covetous-free:

Complete each Scripture below using the New Living Translation.

1. **Accept your** divine **ancestry line.** You are a descendant from a royal line. You are a son/daughter of the Divine Majesty.

    He has made us a _____ of _____ for God his Father. All glory and power to him forever and ever! Amen (Revelation 1:6).

2. **The body is sacred**. You cannot dislike it yet expect your body to work on your behalf. You have to love your body with its physical imperfections. Love is what moves the body to work for you. Look in the mirror every day and compliment yourself. Be the first to tell yourself how beautiful you look. Now, apply this same thought in the spiritual sense. You cannot dislike a particular member of Christ's body; love is needed to grow the Body of Christ. Despite its flaws, you should not speak negatively about a body part or member, for that matter.

    Don't you realize that all of you together are the _____of God and that the _____ of God _____ in you? (1 Corinthians 3:16).

3. **Be truthful to God**. Share with God how you feel, acknowledge your struggles, and release your concerns to Him. He cannot heal until you release.

    Finally, I _____ all my sins to you and stopped trying to _____ my _____. I said to myself, "I will confess my _____ to the LORD." And you forgave me! All my _____ is gone (Psalm 32:5).

4. **Live a disciplined life out of love.** Reward yourself when you step out of the comfort zone. Winning is not always the focus but rather the effort you make to change things.

    No _____ is enjoyable while it is happening—it's painful! But afterward there will be a _____ harvest of right living for those who are _____in this way (Hebrews 12:11).

5. **Forgive yourself.** Christ has forgiven you, so it is your turn to forgive yourself. Live in the present and not in the past. The past can only be revisited if your healing stimulates growth in the other members. Some people's past experiences are powerful testimonies, but the purpose for returning should be to highlight the power of God and not the experience itself.

No, dear brothers and sisters, I have not achieved it, but I focus on this _____ thing: Forgetting the _____ and looking _____ to what lies ahead (Philippians 3:13).

6. **Grow out of the Divine Center.** Your confidence does not spring out of you but out of Christ. Your strength is not from you but from Christ. Your love for self is not from within you but from Christ.

   For _____ comes from him and _____ by his power and is intended for his _____. All glory to him forever! Amen (Romans 11:36).

7. **Acknowledge your Weakness.** Weakness is natural to human existence. We are weak absolutely and relative to God. Acknowledgement of our weakness allows us to experience the power of God.

   Each time he said, "My grace is all you need. My _____ works _____ in _____." So now I am glad to boast about my weaknesses, so that the power of Christ can work through me (2 Corinthians 12:9).

8. **Enjoy yourself**. Cultivate a healthy humor. Laugh at yourself at times.

   A _____ heart is _____ medicine, but a broken spirit _____ a person's strength (Proverbs 17:22).

9. **Eat healthily.** Feed yourself healthy food out of love for it. Your understanding of your body's mission and purpose is the reason you should not put junk in your system. Pour sugar in a car's gas tank and you will eventually kill the engine or cause major damage. Similarly, eat foods that are high in sugar, salt, or fat and you will eventually disable the function of the body.

   Don't be misled—you cannot mock the justice of God. You will always _____ what you _____ (Galatians 6:7).

In an image-driven society, comparison is so tempting and so subtle at times. Sometimes we are not aware that we are comparing. The act of coveting can be secretly hidden in the heart but cannot remain incognito for long. Covetousness is a condition of the heart. In order to protect our heart, we should be content and thankful. We should support each other by celebrating, affirming and forgiving one another. As Jesus ate His last supper with His friends, He created a community of love. He said to them, they will know that you are my disciples by the love you have for one another. What a beautiful picture of pure love!

Your Personal Journey Mission Statement

Personal mission statements should provide a framework for your efforts and help define how you'll approach your health and well-being. Now that you have reached the conclusion of this study, it is time to reflect. Taking a step back to reflect will give you needed insight and will encourage you to think about how you will impact the kingdom of God.

Here are some questions to answer:

What do you need to do to be healthy?

_____

_____

_____

How will you do it?

_____

_____

_____

For whom should you do it?

_____

_____

_____

What value will you be bringing?

_____

_____

_____

Write a personal mission statement based on your responses. Remember your goals should be specific and attainable. Don't be vague and aim for something you're unlikely to reach, which will set you up for failure. Outline how you plan to achieve those goals. Just listing your goals is only half the battle. You must consider how you will get there.

Hold yourself accountable by asking a mentor, an accountability partner, or a trusted friend to meet with you monthly to discuss the progress on your personal goals and mission statement.

Form a small group support group. (See Chapter 10 in *The Ten Guiding Lights to Health and Wholeness* Book)

_____

Notes:

1. Easton's Bible Dictionary, s.v., "covetousness," accessed August 28, 2016, http://www.biblestudytools.com/dictionaries/eastons-bible-dictionary/covetousness.html.
2. 1 Thessalonians 5:18.
3. Luke 2:52.
4. Romans 12:2.
5. The International Agency for Research on Cancer (IARC) has classified processed meat as a carcinogen, something that causes cancer. And it has classified red meat as a probable carcinogen, something that probably causes cancer. IARC is the cancer agency of the World Health Organization. Stacy Simon, "World Health Organization Says Processed meat Causes Cancer," accessed August 28, 2016, http://www.cancer.org/cancer/news/world-health-organization-says-processed-meat-causes-cancer.
6. 1 Corinthians 6:15-20.
7. Joshua 1:8.
8. Bible Hub, s.v. "ruach," accessed August 28, 2016, http://biblehub.com/hebrew/7307.htm.
9. Romans 3:23.
10. David Benner, The Gift of Being Yourself: The Sacred Call to Self-Discovery (Downer Grove, IL: InterVarsity Press, 2004), 82.
11. Ephesians 2:10.
12. Romans 5:7-9.
13. Luke 22:14-20 (GNT).
14. 1 Corinthians 11:29-30.
15. 1 Corinthians 11:28.

3 Ways to Become Physically and Spiritually Fit

1. Cardio:

It is important to exercise daily. The heart is a muscle that requires aerobic type of exercises. No or little exercise can result in cardiovascular diseases and obesity.

Spiritual Parallel: Prayer

No or little prayer will result in spiritual malnutrition or worldly obesity. Remember blessed are those who hunger and thirst after righteousness—"those who *actively* seek right standing with God], for they will be [completely] satisfied" (Matthew 5: 6 AMP). Stay hungry and thirsty for God. We have been called to be distinct from the world in our desires, motives, and outlook of life: "But you are chosen people, royal priests, a holy nation, a people for God's own possession" (I Peter 2:9, NCV). Jesus said of His followers, "They don't belong to the world, just as I don't belong to the world" (John 17:16, NCV).

This type of spiritual exercise must be done daily in order to accomplish spiritual fitness.

What exercise is to the body is what prayer is to the spirit being.

2. Weight-bearing exercises:

The body has two main energy systems: aerobic and anaerobic. Whereas the efficiency of the aerobic system is affiliated with the heart, the anaerobic system is connected with the muscles especially in activities such as weight training. Resistance training should be an integral part of our life. After the age of 25, we lose more than one-half pound of muscle every year. Imagine a house. Your body is like a house. Weight training helps to sustain the structure.

Spiritual Parallel: Adversity/Hardship/Struggles

Adversity builds spiritual muscle. The spiritual muscle that is built is called character: "We also have joy with our troubles, because we know that these troubles produce patience. And patience produces character, and character produces hope" (Romans 5:3-4, NCV).

Adversity, then, is a stepping stone to a higher level. It is progress in the making. But, so many times this is not our outlook. We do not see the pressures in life or the weights we must bear in life as means of refining us in order to become better individuals. If we do not learn to confront the struggles in life by applying the Word of God and see them as opportunities to become stronger, we become flabby Christians.

Adversity is the opportunity to discover the greatness within.

3. Stretching

Stretching is a necessary component of fitness. It increases physical efficiency and performance. It improves muscular balance and postural awareness.

Spiritual Parallel: Faith

When we are challenged in life, our faith is also. We are stretched to surpass our present condition. God stretches us when we allow Him to dream through us. If we are able to accomplish a task all by ourselves, our faith is not stretched. Our faith is stretched when we look to God to achieve the dreams He births in us: With God's power working in us, God can do much, much more than anything we can ask or imagine (Ephesian 3:20, NCV).

Dare to allow God to dream through you.

About the Author

Etta Dale Hornsteiner is the editor of LiveLiving's magazine, which was first published in digital format in 2009. The magazine has become the perfect place for Etta Dale to display her *joi de vivre* and share all the things that inspire her: God and the sacred; holistic health and wellness; athletic discipline; and, theatre and film. The magazine is imbued with the many skills Etta Dale has acquired through the various phases of her life journey.

Etta Dale taught English and Theater for 13 years in the United States and The Bahamas. She competed for seven years as a bodybuilder. It was this fruitful attempt to sculpt the human body that intensified Etta's love for fitness. She left the classroom to become a personal trainer. Helping people whether as a teacher or trainer was the simplest way Etta Dale could respond to the yearning within her heart to see the body of Christ healthy and whole.

Strangely, it was through bodybuilding that she learned the many ways of sculpting not only her body but her spirit and mind as well. She captures these lessons in a unique health and wellness study, *The Ten Guiding Lights to Health and Wellness.* The study underscores the importance of integrating body, mind and spirit to cultivate good physical, mental and spiritual habits for whole health and wellness.

However, it was in meeting and working with Dr. David Allen, a distinguished psychiatrist, that Etta Dale further developed an understanding of the emotional and mental components in order to fully integrate these areas. Etta Dale worked with Dr. Allen in the fine tuning of the Contemplative Discovery Pathway Theory (CDPT), which motivates persons to move beyond their hurt, pain and shame to experience the discovery of their authentic self-based in love and gratitude.

Etta Dale has a strong desire to see people healthy in their body, mind and spirit.

Etta Dale is a graduate of Acadia University in Nova Scotia, Canada with a Bachelor of Arts degree with honors in English and minors in Sociology and Spanish. She received her graduate degree in Education and Theater from Regent University in Virginia Beach, Virginia.

To learn more about Etta Dale's work and to join her e-mail list regarding training and events, visit www.liveliving.org.

Appendix A

TIME	FEELING(S) BEFORE EATING	WHAT I ATE	AMOUNT	FEELING(S) AFTER EATING
MEAL ONE				
MEAL TWO				
MEAL THREE				
MEAL FOUR				
MEAL FIVE				

Appendix B

TIME	FEELING(S) BEFORE EATING	WHAT I ATE	AMOUNT	WATER	PROTEIN (MEAT, BEANS, NUTS)	VEGETABLES	FRUITS	GRAINS	FAT	FEELING(S) AFTER EATING
MEAL ONE										
MEAL TWO										
MEAL THREE										
MEAL FOUR										
MEAL FIVE										

Appendix C

WORKOUT LOG

DATE:	WEEK:
MONDAY	

EXERCISE NAME	DISTANCE/ TIME/ SETS/ REPS

DATE:	WEEK:
TUESDAY	

EXERCISE NAME	DISTANCE/ TIME/ SETS/ REPS

DATE:	WEEK:
WEDNESDAY	

EXERCISE NAME	DISTANCE/ TIME/ SETS/ REPS

DATE:	WEEK:
THURSDAY	

EXERCISE NAME	DISTANCE/ TIME/ SETS/ REPS

DATE:	WEEK:
FRIDAY	

EXERCISE NAME	DISTANCE/ TIME/ SETS/ REPS

DATE:	WEEK:
SATURDAY/SUNDAY	

EXERCISE NAME	DISTANCE/ TIME/ SETS/ REPS

Bibliography

Ankrom, S. *Very Well*, "Neurotransmitters: The Chemical Messengers of the Brain," accessed May 5, 2016,
https://www.verywell.com/neurotransmitters-description-and-categories-2584400.

THE
TEN GUIDING LIGHTS
TO HEALTH
AND
WHOLENESS

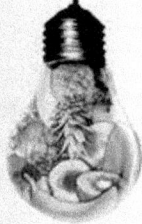

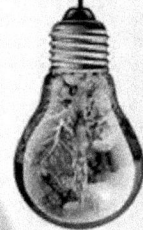

ETTA D. HORNSTEINER

The Ten Guiding Lights to Health and Wholeness
Learn how taking care of your body can aid you on your spiritual journey.

Available on Amazon and through your local book store.

IISBN: 978-0-9985096-0-0

For more information visit liveliving.org

* 9 7 8 0 9 9 8 5 0 9 6 1 7 *

Key Control Log

COMPANY DETAILS

COMPANY NAME

ADDRESS

E-MAIL ADDRESS

WEBSITE

PHONE   **FAX**

EMERGENCY CONTACT PERSON

PHONE   **FAX**

LOG BOOK DETAILS

CONTINUED FROM LOG BOOK

LOG START DATE

CONTINUED TO LOG BOOK

LOG END DATE

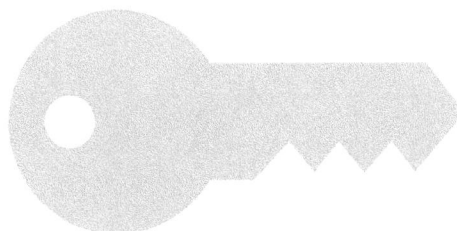

Dedication

This Key Control Log Book is dedicated to all the businesses out there who want to keep track and record who has what key and document their findings in the process.

You are my inspiration for producing books and I'm honored to be a part of keeping all of your key notes and records organized.

This journal notebook will help you record the details of your key control.

Thoughtfully put together with these sections to record: Period, Department, Key No., Time & Date Signed Out, Signed Out Name & Signature, Time & Date Returned, & Returned By Signature.

How to Use this Book

The purpose of this book is to keep all of your Key Control notes all in one place. It will help keep you organized.

This Key Control Log Book will allow you to accurately document every detail about your key control.

Here are examples of the prompts for you to fill in and write about your experience in this book:

1. Period

2. Department

3. Key Number

4. Time & Date Signed Out

5. Signed Out Name

6. Signed Out Signature

7. Time & Date Returned

8. Returned By Name & Sign

Key Control Log

PERIOD   **DEPARTMENT**

Key No.	Time & Date Signed Out	Signed Out Name	Signed Out Signature	Time & Date Returned	Returned by Name & Sign

Key Control Log

PERIOD   **DEPARTMENT**

Key No.	Time & Date Signed Out	Signed Out Name	Signed Out Signature	Time & Date Returned	Returned by Name & Sign

Key Control Log

PERIOD   **DEPARTMENT**

Key No.	Time & Date Signed Out	Signed Out Name	Signed Out Signature	Time & Date Returned	Returned by Name & Sign

Key Control Log

PERIOD   DEPARTMENT

Key No.	Time & Date Signed Out	Signed Out Name	Signed Out Signature	Time & Date Returned	Returned by Name & Sign

Key Control Log

PERIOD   **DEPARTMENT**

Key No.	Time & Date Signed Out	Signed Out Name	Signed Out Signature	Time & Date Returned	Returned by Name & Sign

Key Control Log

PERIOD   **DEPARTMENT**

Key No.	Time & Date Signed Out	Signed Out Name	Signed Out Signature	Time & Date Returned	Returned by Name & Sign

Key Control Log

PERIOD _____   **DEPARTMENT**

Key No.	Time & Date Signed Out	Signed Out Name	Signed Out Signature	Time & Date Returned	Returned by Name & Sign

Key Control Log

PERIOD   **DEPARTMENT**

Key No.	Time & Date Signed Out	Signed Out Name	Signed Out Signature	Time & Date Returned	Returned by Name & Sign

Key Control Log

PERIOD   DEPARTMENT

Key No.	Time & Date Signed Out	Signed Out Name	Signed Out Signature	Time & Date Returned	Returned by Name & Sign

Key Control Log

PERIOD   **DEPARTMENT**

Key No.	Time & Date Signed Out	Signed Out Name	Signed Out Signature	Time & Date Returned	Returned by Name & Sign

Key Control Log

PERIOD   **DEPARTMENT**

Key No.	Time & Date Signed Out	Signed Out Name	Signed Out Signature	Time & Date Returned	Returned by Name & Sign

Key Control Log

PERIOD **DEPARTMENT**

Key No.	Time & Date Signed Out	Signed Out Name	Signed Out Signature	Time & Date Returned	Returned by Name & Sign

Key Control Log

         DEPARTMENT

Key No.	Time & Date Signed Out	Signed Out Name	Signed Out Signature	Time & Date Returned	Returned by Name & Sign

Key Control Log

PERIOD   **DEPARTMENT**

Key No.	Time & Date Signed Out	Signed Out Name	Signed Out Signature	Time & Date Returned	Returned by Name & Sign

Key Control Log

PERIOD   **DEPARTMENT**

Key No.	Time & Date Signed Out	Signed Out Name	Signed Out Signature	Time & Date Returned	Returned by Name & Sign

Key Control Log

PERIOD   DEPARTMENT

Key No.	Time & Date Signed Out	Signed Out Name	Signed Out Signature	Time & Date Returned	Returned by Name & Sign

Key Control Log

PERIOD _____ **DEPARTMENT** _____

Key No.	Time & Date Signed Out	Signed Out Name	Signed Out Signature	Time & Date Returned	Returned by Name & Sign

Key Control Log

PERIOD   **DEPARTMENT**

Key No.	Time & Date Signed Out	Signed Out Name	Signed Out Signature	Time & Date Returned	Returned by Name & Sign

Key Control Log

PERIOD   DEPARTMENT

Key No.	Time & Date Signed Out	Signed Out Name	Signed Out Signature	Time & Date Returned	Returned by Name & Sign

Key Control Log

PERIOD   DEPARTMENT

Key No.	Time & Date Signed Out	Signed Out Name	Signed Out Signature	Time & Date Returned	Returned by Name & Sign

Key Control Log

PERIOD   **DEPARTMENT**

Key No.	Time & Date Signed Out	Signed Out Name	Signed Out Signature	Time & Date Returned	Returned by Name & Sign

Key Control Log

PERIOD   **DEPARTMENT**

Key No.	Time & Date Signed Out	Signed Out Name	Signed Out Signature	Time & Date Returned	Returned by Name & Sign

Key Control Log

PERIOD   **DEPARTMENT**

Key No.	Time & Date Signed Out	Signed Out Name	Signed Out Signature	Time & Date Returned	Returned by Name & Sign

Key Control Log

PERIOD   **DEPARTMENT**

Key No.	Time & Date Signed Out	Signed Out Name	Signed Out Signature	Time & Date Returned	Returned by Name & Sign

Key Control Log

PERIOD   **DEPARTMENT**

Key No.	Time & Date Signed Out	Signed Out Name	Signed Out Signature	Time & Date Returned	Returned by Name & Sign

Key Control Log

PERIOD   **DEPARTMENT**

Key No.	Time & Date Signed Out	Signed Out Name	Signed Out Signature	Time & Date Returned	Returned by Name & Sign

Key Control Log

PERIOD   **DEPARTMENT**

Key No.	Time & Date Signed Out	Signed Out Name	Signed Out Signature	Time & Date Returned	Returned by Name & Sign

Key Control Log

PERIOD   **DEPARTMENT**

Key No.	Time & Date Signed Out	Signed Out Name	Signed Out Signature	Time & Date Returned	Returned by Name & Sign

Key Control Log

PERIOD   **DEPARTMENT**

Key No.	Time & Date Signed Out	Signed Out Name	Signed Out Signature	Time & Date Returned	Returned by Name & Sign

Key Control Log

PERIOD   **DEPARTMENT**

Key No.	Time & Date Signed Out	Signed Out Name	Signed Out Signature	Time & Date Returned	Returned by Name & Sign

Key Control Log

       DEPARTMENT

Key No.	Time & Date Signed Out	Signed Out Name	Signed Out Signature	Time & Date Returned	Returned by Name & Sign

Key Control Log

PERIOD **DEPARTMENT**

Key No.	Time & Date Signed Out	Signed Out Name	Signed Out Signature	Time & Date Returned	Returned by Name & Sign

Key Control Log

PERIOD   **DEPARTMENT**

Key No.	Time & Date Signed Out	Signed Out Name	Signed Out Signature	Time & Date Returned	Returned by Name & Sign

Key Control Log

PERIOD   **DEPARTMENT**

Key No.	Time & Date Signed Out	Signed Out Name	Signed Out Signature	Time & Date Returned	Returned by Name & Sign

Key Control Log

PERIOD _____   **DEPARTMENT** _____

Key No.	Time & Date Signed Out	Signed Out Name	Signed Out Signature	Time & Date Returned	Returned by Name & Sign

Key Control Log

PERIOD   **DEPARTMENT**

Key No.	Time & Date Signed Out	Signed Out Name	Signed Out Signature	Time & Date Returned	Returned by Name & Sign

Key Control Log

PERIOD   **DEPARTMENT**

Key No.	Time & Date Signed Out	Signed Out Name	Signed Out Signature	Time & Date Returned	Returned by Name & Sign

Key Control Log

PERIOD   **DEPARTMENT**

Key No.	Time & Date Signed Out	Signed Out Name	Signed Out Signature	Time & Date Returned	Returned by Name & Sign

Key Control Log

PERIOD _____   **DEPARTMENT** _____

Key No.	Time & Date Signed Out	Signed Out Name	Signed Out Signature	Time & Date Returned	Returned by Name & Sign

Key Control Log

PERIOD **DEPARTMENT**

Key No.	Time & Date Signed Out	Signed Out Name	Signed Out Signature	Time & Date Returned	Returned by Name & Sign

Key Control Log

PERIOD   **DEPARTMENT**

Key No.	Time & Date Signed Out	Signed Out Name	Signed Out Signature	Time & Date Returned	Returned by Name & Sign

Key Control Log

PERIOD   **DEPARTMENT**

Key No.	Time & Date Signed Out	Signed Out Name	Signed Out Signature	Time & Date Returned	Returned by Name & Sign

Key Control Log

PERIOD _____ **DEPARTMENT** _____

Key No.	Time & Date Signed Out	Signed Out Name	Signed Out Signature	Time & Date Returned	Returned by Name & Sign

Key Control Log

PERIOD _____   DEPARTMENT _____

Key No.	Time & Date Signed Out	Signed Out Name	Signed Out Signature	Time & Date Returned	Returned by Name & Sign

Key Control Log

PERIOD   **DEPARTMENT**

Key No.	Time & Date Signed Out	Signed Out Name	Signed Out Signature	Time & Date Returned	Returned by Name & Sign

Key Control Log

PERIOD   **DEPARTMENT**

Key No.	Time & Date Signed Out	Signed Out Name	Signed Out Signature	Time & Date Returned	Returned by Name & Sign

Key Control Log

PERIOD **DEPARTMENT**

Key No.	Time & Date Signed Out	Signed Out Name	Signed Out Signature	Time & Date Returned	Returned by Name & Sign

Key Control Log

PERIOD   **DEPARTMENT**

Key No.	Time & Date Signed Out	Signed Out Name	Signed Out Signature	Time & Date Returned	Returned by Name & Sign

Key Control Log

PERIOD   DEPARTMENT

Key No.	Time & Date Signed Out	Signed Out Name	Signed Out Signature	Time & Date Returned	Returned by Name & Sign

Key Control Log

PERIOD   **DEPARTMENT**

Key No.	Time & Date Signed Out	Signed Out Name	Signed Out Signature	Time & Date Returned	Returned by Name & Sign

Key Control Log

PERIOD　　　　　　　　　　**DEPARTMENT**

Key No.	Time & Date Signed Out	Signed Out Name	Signed Out Signature	Time & Date Returned	Returned by Name & Sign

Key Control Log

PERIOD   **DEPARTMENT**

Key No.	Time & Date Signed Out	Signed Out Name	Signed Out Signature	Time & Date Returned	Returned by Name & Sign

Key Control Log

PERIOD   **DEPARTMENT**

Key No.	Time & Date Signed Out	Signed Out Name	Signed Out Signature	Time & Date Returned	Returned by Name & Sign

Key Control Log

PERIOD   **DEPARTMENT**

Key No.	Time & Date Signed Out	Signed Out Name	Signed Out Signature	Time & Date Returned	Returned by Name & Sign

Key Control Log

PERIOD   **DEPARTMENT**

Key No.	Time & Date Signed Out	Signed Out Name	Signed Out Signature	Time & Date Returned	Returned by Name & Sign

Key Control Log

PERIOD   **DEPARTMENT**

Key No.	Time & Date Signed Out	Signed Out Name	Signed Out Signature	Time & Date Returned	Returned by Name & Sign

Key Control Log

PERIOD _____   **DEPARTMENT** _____

Key No.	Time & Date Signed Out	Signed Out Name	Signed Out Signature	Time & Date Returned	Returned by Name & Sign

Key Control Log

PERIOD   **DEPARTMENT**

Key No.	Time & Date Signed Out	Signed Out Name	Signed Out Signature	Time & Date Returned	Returned by Name & Sign

Key Control Log

PERIOD   **DEPARTMENT**

Key No.	Time & Date Signed Out	Signed Out Name	Signed Out Signature	Time & Date Returned	Returned by Name & Sign

Key Control Log

PERIOD   **DEPARTMENT**

Key No.	Time & Date Signed Out	Signed Out Name	Signed Out Signature	Time & Date Returned	Returned by Name & Sign

Key Control Log

PERIOD   **DEPARTMENT**

Key No.	Time & Date Signed Out	Signed Out Name	Signed Out Signature	Time & Date Returned	Returned by Name & Sign

Key Control Log

PERIOD _____ **DEPARTMENT** _____

Key No.	Time & Date Signed Out	Signed Out Name	Signed Out Signature	Time & Date Returned	Returned by Name & Sign

Key Control Log

PERIOD   **DEPARTMENT**

Key No.	Time & Date Signed Out	Signed Out Name	Signed Out Signature	Time & Date Returned	Returned by Name & Sign

Key Control Log

PERIOD _____   DEPARTMENT _____

Key No.	Time & Date Signed Out	Signed Out Name	Signed Out Signature	Time & Date Returned	Returned by Name & Sign

Key Control Log

PERIOD   **DEPARTMENT**

Key No.	Time & Date Signed Out	Signed Out Name	Signed Out Signature	Time & Date Returned	Returned by Name & Sign

Key Control Log

PERIOD   **DEPARTMENT**

Key No.	Time & Date Signed Out	Signed Out Name	Signed Out Signature	Time & Date Returned	Returned by Name & Sign

Key Control Log

PERIOD _____ **DEPARTMENT** _____

Key No.	Time & Date Signed Out	Signed Out Name	Signed Out Signature	Time & Date Returned	Returned by Name & Sign

Key Control Log

PERIOD   DEPARTMENT

Key No.	Time & Date Signed Out	Signed Out Name	Signed Out Signature	Time & Date Returned	Returned by Name & Sign

Key Control Log

PERIOD _____   **DEPARTMENT** _____

Key No.	Time & Date Signed Out	Signed Out Name	Signed Out Signature	Time & Date Returned	Returned by Name & Sign

Key Control Log

PERIOD _____ **DEPARTMENT** _____

Key No.	Time & Date Signed Out	Signed Out Name	Signed Out Signature	Time & Date Returned	Returned by Name & Sign

Key Control Log

PERIOD   **DEPARTMENT**

Key No.	Time & Date Signed Out	Signed Out Name	Signed Out Signature	Time & Date Returned	Returned by Name & Sign

Key Control Log

PERIOD　　　　　　　　**DEPARTMENT**

Key No.	Time & Date Signed Out	Signed Out Name	Signed Out Signature	Time & Date Returned	Returned by Name & Sign

Key Control Log

PERIOD　　　　　　　　　　　**DEPARTMENT**

Key No.	Time & Date Signed Out	Signed Out Name	Signed Out Signature	Time & Date Returned	Returned by Name & Sign

Key Control Log

PERIOD   **DEPARTMENT**

Key No.	Time & Date Signed Out	Signed Out Name	Signed Out Signature	Time & Date Returned	Returned by Name & Sign

Key Control Log

PERIOD   **DEPARTMENT**

Key No.	Time & Date Signed Out	Signed Out Name	Signed Out Signature	Time & Date Returned	Returned by Name & Sign

Key Control Log

PERIOD   **DEPARTMENT**

Key No.	Time & Date Signed Out	Signed Out Name	Signed Out Signature	Time & Date Returned	Returned by Name & Sign

Key Control Log

PERIOD   **DEPARTMENT**

Key No.	Time & Date Signed Out	Signed Out Name	Signed Out Signature	Time & Date Returned	Returned by Name & Sign

Key Control Log

PERIOD   DEPARTMENT

Key No.	Time & Date Signed Out	Signed Out Name	Signed Out Signature	Time & Date Returned	Returned by Name & Sign

Key Control Log

PERIOD   **DEPARTMENT**

Key No.	Time & Date Signed Out	Signed Out Name	Signed Out Signature	Time & Date Returned	Returned by Name & Sign

Key Control Log

PERIOD   DEPARTMENT

Key No.	Time & Date Signed Out	Signed Out Name	Signed Out Signature	Time & Date Returned	Returned by Name & Sign

Key Control Log

PERIOD   **DEPARTMENT**

Key No.	Time & Date Signed Out	Signed Out Name	Signed Out Signature	Time & Date Returned	Returned by Name & Sign

Key Control Log

PERIOD   **DEPARTMENT**

Key No.	Time & Date Signed Out	Signed Out Name	Signed Out Signature	Time & Date Returned	Returned by Name & Sign

Key Control Log

PERIOD   **DEPARTMENT**

Key No.	Time & Date Signed Out	Signed Out Name	Signed Out Signature	Time & Date Returned	Returned by Name & Sign

Key Control Log

PERIOD   **DEPARTMENT**

Key No.	Time & Date Signed Out	Signed Out Name	Signed Out Signature	Time & Date Returned	Returned by Name & Sign

Key Control Log

PERIOD　　　　　　　　　　**DEPARTMENT**

Key No.	Time & Date Signed Out	Signed Out Name	Signed Out Signature	Time & Date Returned	Returned by Name & Sign

Key Control Log

PERIOD   **DEPARTMENT**

Key No.	Time & Date Signed Out	Signed Out Name	Signed Out Signature	Time & Date Returned	Returned by Name & Sign

Key Control Log

PERIOD

DEPARTMENT

Key No.	Time & Date Signed Out	Signed Out Name	Signed Out Signature	Time & Date Returned	Returned by Name & Sign

Key Control Log

PERIOD   **DEPARTMENT**

Key No.	Time & Date Signed Out	Signed Out Name	Signed Out Signature	Time & Date Returned	Returned by Name & Sign

Key Control Log

PERIOD   **DEPARTMENT**

Key No.	Time & Date Signed Out	Signed Out Name	Signed Out Signature	Time & Date Returned	Returned by Name & Sign

Key Control Log

PERIOD   **DEPARTMENT**

Key No.	Time & Date Signed Out	Signed Out Name	Signed Out Signature	Time & Date Returned	Returned by Name & Sign

Key Control Log

PERIOD   **DEPARTMENT**

Key No.	Time & Date Signed Out	Signed Out Name	Signed Out Signature	Time & Date Returned	Returned by Name & Sign

Key Control Log

PERIOD   **DEPARTMENT**

Key No.	Time & Date Signed Out	Signed Out Name	Signed Out Signature	Time & Date Returned	Returned by Name & Sign

Key Control Log

PERIOD _____   **DEPARTMENT** _____

Key No.	Time & Date Signed Out	Signed Out Name	Signed Out Signature	Time & Date Returned	Returned by Name & Sign

Key Control Log

PERIOD   **DEPARTMENT**

Key No.	Time & Date Signed Out	Signed Out Name	Signed Out Signature	Time & Date Returned	Returned by Name & Sign

Key Control Log

PERIOD

DEPARTMENT

Key No.	Time & Date Signed Out	Signed Out Name	Signed Out Signature	Time & Date Returned	Returned by Name & Sign

Key Control Log

PERIOD   DEPARTMENT

Key No.	Time & Date Signed Out	Signed Out Name	Signed Out Signature	Time & Date Returned	Returned by Name & Sign

Key Control Log

PERIOD   **DEPARTMENT**

Key No.	Time & Date Signed Out	Signed Out Name	Signed Out Signature	Time & Date Returned	Returned by Name & Sign

www.ingramcontent.com/pod-product-compliance
Lightning Source LLC
Chambersburg PA
CBHW080349050426
42336CB00053B/3286